THE ESSENTIAL GUIDE TO
OILS

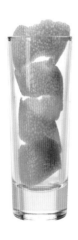

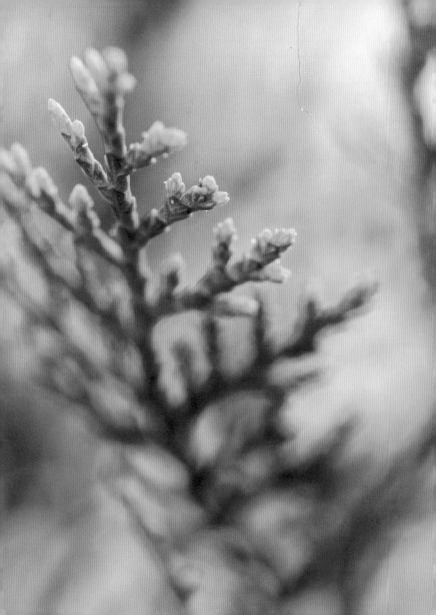

THE ESSENTIAL GUIDE TO
OILS

**ALL THE HEALING OILS YOU WILL EVER
NEED FOR WELL-BEING AND VITALITY**

JENNIE HARDING

WATKINS PUBLISHING
LONDON

This edition first published in the UK
and USA in 2013 by
Watkins Publishing Limited
PO Box 883
Oxford, OX1 9PL, UK

A member of Osprey Group

A CIP record for this book is available
from the British Library

ISBN: 978-1-78028-516-0

10 9 8 7 6 5 4 3 2

Typeset in GillSans
Colour reproduction by XY Digital
Printed in China

Publisher's Note: The information
in this book is not intended as a
substitute for professional medical
advice and treatment. If you are
pregnant or suffering from any health
problems, you should consult a medical
professional before following any of
the advice suggested here. Watkins
Publishing Ltd, or any persons involved
in creating this publication, cannot
accept responsibility for any injuries or
damage incurred as a result of following the information presented.

Watkins Publishing is supporting the
Woodland Trust, the UK's leading
woodland conservation charity,
by funding tree-planting initiatives and
woodland maintenance.

watkinspublishing.co.uk

Contents

Introduction

Welcome to the world of essential oils, and a journey that will take you beyond the commercial fragrances you encounter every day to the powerful, natural aromas hidden within plants. These are the same aromas that draw bees to flowers, or that call out to you and make you stop by a bush of scented roses so that the gentle softness can envelop your senses. They are the actual fragrances of Nature; and they make you breathe in, sigh and relax.

When we react to these natural aromas, we respond to the fragrance that comes from a plant's essential oil, a precious liquid that can be extracted and then used in aromatherapy. The aromas of essential oils evaporate much more quickly than the chemical-laden, synthetic aromas of cosmetic perfumes, which is why their scent is deeper, richer and more powerful. In addition, essential oils have specific, healing effects on mind and body that commercial oils do not have. Oils such as Rose Absolute can cause both your mind and body to relax deeply, while those such as Eucalyptus can help you to breathe more easily, and others such as Lemon can boost your immune system. The profound inner healing effects of these and hundreds of other essential oils make aromatherapy one of the most effective tools to soothe physical and emotional stress, too.

Over time, humankind has discovered how to use special techniques, such as steam distillation, to extract essential oils from plants so that we can use them directly. This has led to the development of holistic aromatherapy, a gentle approach to healing the mind, body and spirit with essential oils. Holistic aromatherapy is aromatherapy in its truest sense: blends aren't ready-made or off-the-shelf, but carefully combined by a qualified practitioner to heal the "whole" person, according to his or her symptoms and smell preferences.

In this book we cover 88 essential oils and 12 carrier oils. Many essential oils, such as Lavender and Peppermint, are easy to obtain, while others, such as Rose Otto and Melissa, are rare. Learning to become a connoisseur of essential oils is rather like developing a nose for fine wine: it comes with practice. This book will start you on your way, demonstrating the wonderful versatility and effects of the oils. You will discover how to choose essential oils, how to store them and how to use them safely and effectively for your own well-being.

Over my 16 years of aromatherapy practice, I have noticed that people respond to essential oils because they remind them of Nature. Modern life separates us from the Earth, its cycles and seasons. Sitting in cars or behind computers, and spending hours in offices away from natural light all dampen the spirit. For millennia, our ancestors spent most of their time outdoors, finding food, perfumes and medicine, leading a way of life that was much more in tune with Nature. Plants have a unique link to humankind: they have been tasted, smelled, picked and used throughout our history. Aromatic plants have a particular appeal, explaining why many of them have become integral to our gardens, and used in cooking as flavours, or in perfumes, ointments and oils to anoint the body. All thanks to their essential oils – the source of their fragrance.

I first opened a bottle of essential oil more than twenty years ago. I didn't know anything about aromatherapy; I simply picked up a bottle labelled "Lavender" and took off the lid. The aroma filled the space, and I was amazed by how it soothed me. This act changed my life: I went on to study aromatherapy and make it my career. Since then, my journey with essential oils has been profound. Now I wish you well on your own path of aromatic discovery.

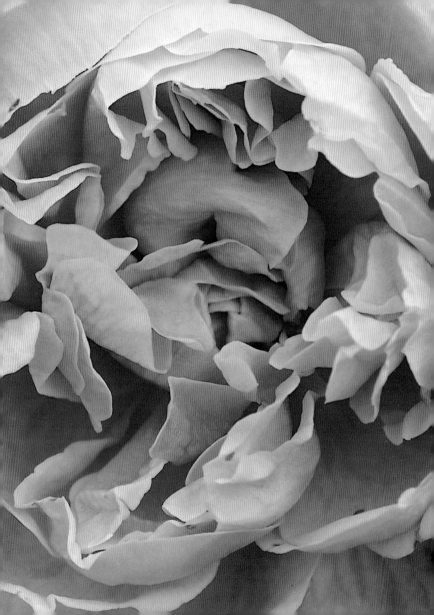

Part One:
The Power of Essential Oils

This section marks the beginning of your voyage of discovery – your first step into the wonderful world of essential oils. On these pages you will learn what essential oils are, where they come from, how they are produced and how they work on the body, mind and spirit to improve health, vitality and well-being. You'll learn how to harness the amazing power of your sense of smell and use it to experience profound relaxation. You'll unearth the many versatile ways in which to integrate essential oils into your daily life. And you'll learn about how to use essential oils safely, enabling you to get the best out of aromatherapy, in the most positive and supportive ways for you.

What is aromatherapy?

Aromatherapy is the specific use of the natural fragrances of the essential oils in aromatic plants to enhance physical, mental and emotional well-being. Using aromatic substances – by inhaling them, applying them in massage or via many other techniques – is not new: since ancient times, civilizations all over the world have valued fragrant plants, flowers, woods and resins for their healing powers and their relaxing and uplifting effects on the mind. The Ancient Egyptians, for example, used frankincense resin on a massive scale, burning it as incense to purify sacred space in temples and in the living quarters of the pharaohs; as well as using it in perfumes, skincare preparations, wound-healing and embalming. In India, for thousands of years, aromas from flowers such as jasmine and rose, from woods such as sandalwood, and from herbs such as patchouli have had a multitude of uses – in aromatic, floral garlands draped around statues, in incense blends, in oil-based perfumes and in skincare.

Essential oils – their first uses

Aromatherapy as we know it today is a different approach from these early beginnings, because it requires the extraction of essential oils from natural plant materials, rather than using the plant materials themselves. Nevertheless, the main production technique for essential oils – distillation – is at least hundreds of years old, emerging in Europe, thanks to the Arab civilizations, in the early part of the tenth century CE (see p.18). In western Europe, essential oils have been used in perfumery since the 16th century, when the German scientist Hieronymus von Braunschweig wrote the first technical manual on distillation. "Eau de Cologne", for example, which was created in the 18th century, contained the distilled essential oils of Orange, Lemon, Rosemary, Lavender and Bergamot. Oils have also been used medicinally for hundreds of years. In France, Italy and Germany, in the late-19th century, certain oils provided early antibiotics. During World War I essential oils such as Rosemary and Tea Tree were used in hospitals as natural antiseptics and wound-healers.

Aromatherapy – a developing art

Aromatherapy as a therapeutic practice did not emerge until the early 20th century. One of its founding fathers, in the 1930s, was French perfumer René Maurice Gattefosse. He treated a burn on his hand with Lavender oil and was astonished at how quickly it healed. Realizing from this that essential oils had therapeutic as well as fragrant potential, he coined the name "aroma*therapy*". Through the work of other pioneers, such as Austrian-born Marguerite Maury in the 1960s, who came up with the idea of massage application, and Britain's Robert Tisserand, who published the first book on aromatherapy in the 1970s, aromatherapy gradually became the practice we know today.

Aromatherapy practice varies according to which country you live in. In the UK, other parts of Europe, Australasia, Canada and the Far East, trained aromatherapists study physiology, massage techniques and the properties of essential oils, enabling them to make blends tailored to clients' specific needs. In the US, regulations vary, but registered massage practitioners are often wary of legal constraints, so most will use pre-prepared commercial blends of oils. If you are looking for an aromatherapy treatment, always consult a professional body in your country to find a qualified practitioner (see p.278).

What aromatherapy can do

Accessibility is one of the most wonderful things about aromatherapy. You could go out today, buy some essential oils and start using them straightaway. Even something as simple as using two drops of Lavender oil on your pillow at night to help you to sleep is aromatherapy – the gentle aroma helps to relieve tension and improve relaxation, so that your sleep is more restful.

Relieving stress and burnout

The most important benefit of aromatherapy is stress-relief. Sadly, for many people, stress is a fact of modern life – a combination of work and family pressures and financial and environmental issues propels us toward burnout. The good news is that aromatherapy can help us to relax. Often, a scent will make us feel calmer immediately, for no apparent reason; but sometimes the scent of a particular oil will remind us of childhood or of times in our lives when we felt more at ease. When we use this type of oil in aromatherapy, the former relaxed state is recaptured by the memory that the scent triggers.

Many people turn to aromatherapy to be "energized". While some oils do have an energizing effect on parts of the body, such as Rosemary on the muscles or Mandarin on the mind, aromatherapy's deepest benefit lies not in stimulation, but rather in *restoration* – bringing back balance to mind, body and spirit. Indeed, when we are exhausted, an overstimulated body doesn't need energizing, it needs harmonizing. Essential oils bring a sense of deep calm, and aromatherapy gives us quality "time out", during which we can allow the body to recover from stress – and, in time, feel re-energized. In the long term, this has invaluable benefits for our overall well-being.

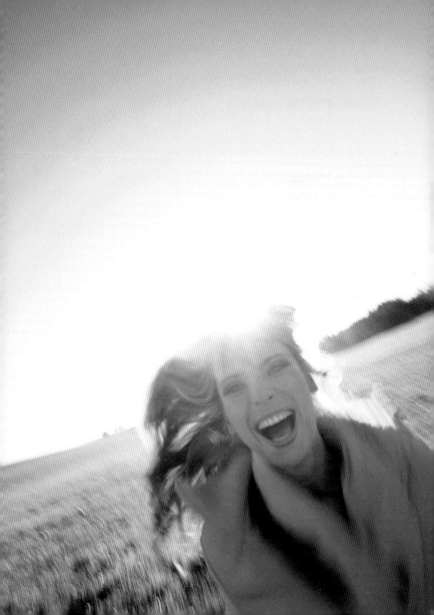

What is an essential oil?

Essential oils are potent liquids that form as part of the internal structure of aromatic plants. In certain parts of these plants, special microscopic sacs gradually fill up with the oil as the plant matures. One of the easiest ways to see this is to pare off an extremely thin piece of orange rind and then look at the underside. You should see hundreds of tiny circular globes, which are the essential oil sacs in the peel. Grating the zest or pressing it with a nail will burst them open, releasing the tangy orange fragrance – the essential oil.

The source of nature's ingenious aromas

The sacs of essential oil appear in differing parts of different plants. In citrus fruits the oil comes from the peel (see above). Some plants, such as scented geraniums or patchouli, produce thousands of silky hairs on the upper surface of their leaves, at the end of which are special cells filled with essential oil. Rubbing the surface of these leaves therefore feels sticky and results in a strong aroma on your fingers. Leaves are also the source of the many essential oils that come from common herbs, such as rosemary and basil. (A lot of these plants thrive in the Mediterranean sunshine, producing particularly high amounts of oil inside the leaves.) Flowers such as lavender, rose and jasmine produce oil in their petals. The oil is concentrated toward the centre of the flower to attract pollinators such as butterflies and bees. Other essential oils are found in wood, such as the oil from Himalayan cedar, or in roots, such as that from ginger. These oils protect the tree or plant from attack by tiny predators by making the tissues of the plant smell unattractive to insects – although, of course, humans often love the very same smells!

A varied palette

Most essential oils are colourless liquids. The exceptions are Yarrow, German
Chamomile, Vetiver and Spikenard. Yarrow and German Chamomile are
bright blue, as these oils contain a special deep blue, aromatic compound
called azulene. Vetiver, which comes from the roots of the plant of the
same name, is dark brown and sticky. Spikenard, also from its plant's roots,
is green. In addition, absolutes, such as Rose or Jasmine, which are produced
by a chemical process (see p.18), tend to be deep yellow or orange, as they
contain traces of the plant pigments that gave the original petals their colour.
However, none of these coloured oils will colour your skin. In fact, when they
are made into blends (see pp.40–41), the colour dissolves in the carrier oil.

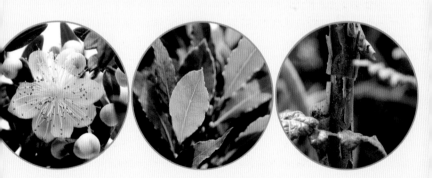

What part of a plant does an essential oil come from? The answer is: it depends on the plant and
the oil you want to extract. Flowers, leaves and bark are among the potential sources.

Essential oils worldwide

One of the most fascinating features of essential oils is their ability to conjure up the atmosphere of exotic places around the world. Open a bottle and you could be smelling Sweet Orange from Brazil, Patchouli from Indonesia or Rose Otto from Bulgaria – the smells are like a magic carpet, transporting you on a sensory journey to every corner of the globe.

A world of fragrance

The aromatic plants that produce essential oils are most commonly found in temperate parts of the world (those with mild winters and hot summers); arid areas (which are dry and desert-like); and sub-tropical and tropical regions (with hot, moist climates). Few flourish in cold regions, an exception being aromatic evergreen trees, such as pine, which grows in northern Europe, the US and Canada.

Europe is a major source of essential oils. Many come from plants that thrive in the hot Mediterranean region of southern Europe. This area is home to the largest essential-oil-rich group of plants of all – classified as the *Labiatae* – which includes lavender, rosemary and peppermint. Citrus trees, such as orange, mandarin and lemon, which originally came from China, also thrive here. Meanwhile, powerful aromatic plants, such as fennel, coriander and angelica, are found growing in central Europe.

In Bulgaria, Turkey and Morocco, damask roses produce Rose Otto, one of the most exquisite essential oils. The deserts of North Africa and the Middle East yield oils from resins, sticky substances that ooze out of damaged tree bark; Frankincense and Myrrh are two famous examples, prized since antiquity for use in incense. Other sources of more exotic essential oils are Indonesia, which produces Patchouli and Vetiver; Madagascar, the home of Ylang Ylang; and India, which is world-famous as a producer of Cardamom, Jasmine and Lemongrass, as well as the classic Indian Sandalwood.

Sandalwood – an endangered resource

One of the most highly prized essential oils, Indian Sandalwood is distilled from the fragrant inner wood of the sandalwood tree (*Santalum album*). These trees take around forty years to mature and to produce oil at full potency. However, they have become endangered in recent times, mainly owing to illegal logging, and there is now a world shortage of quality Indian Sandalwood oil.

As a result, producers have started looking to Australian sandalwood (*Santalum spicatum*), native to Western Australia, for an alternative supply. By managing these trees with care, the Australians are able to offer a sustainable source of essential oil.

Australian Sandalwood oil has a milder fragrance than the Indian form. Its chemical content is different, but it can be used in the same way (see p.208).

17

Producing essential oils

It takes a great deal of plant material to extract essential oils in significant quantities – fields of plants or acres of trees. Farmers know exactly when to harvest the plants for maximum oil yield, and the extraction process is labour- and time-intensive, which is why essential oils are relatively expensive.

Extracting the oils – distillation

In the tenth century CE, the Arabian physician Avicenna is thought to have been the first to use steam distillation to extract aromatic liquids from plants. In the late Renaissance, German and Swiss scientists refined the technique, and today, steam distillation (see diagram, right) remains the main method by which we obtain essential oils. The containers (called "stills") used in distillation can be stainless steel and installed in state-of-the-art factories, or simply oil drums linked to handmade pipes. Distillation begins by placing plant material in the still. In a factory, steam is then pumped through the plant material; for the simpler method, plants are soaked in water and a fire is lit underneath. Either way, the heat lifts the essential oils out of the plant fibres to form a fragrant steam. This is piped to a chamber (a condenser) surrounded by a coil filled with cold water, which cools the steam back to water and leaves the oil floating on the water's surface, from where it can be siphoned off. The remaining water is aromatic, too – it is rose water, lavender water and so on.

Other methods of extraction

• **Solvent extraction:** This is used to make absolutes – highly concentrated, usually floral liquids. Petals are soaked in a chemical solvent so that their

Diagram of steam distillation

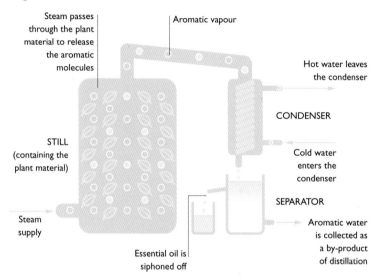

Steam passes through the plant material to release the aromatic molecules

Aromatic vapour

Hot water leaves the condenser

CONDENSER

STILL (containing the plant material)

Cold water enters the condenser

SEPARATOR

Steam supply

Aromatic water is collected as a by-product of distillation

Essential oil is siphoned off

fragrant molecules separate and sink. The solvent is then reprocessed to remove the aromatic residue. Solvent extraction is used for delicate flowers such as jasmine (see pp.260–61), which cannot withstand steam distillation.

- **Expression:** Used to give us citrus oils (such as Mandarin; pp.258–9), this process literally squeezes the oil from the fruit peel of lemons, mandarins, oranges, and so on, preserving all the freshness of the aroma.

Buying and storing essential oils

Always buy quality essential oils from suppliers who source their products carefully. In aromatherapy, quality oils give the best results and are less likely to cause any adverse reactions or to compromise safety (see pp.22–9). Unfortunately, the adulteration and dilution of essential oils (usually by adding petrochemicals to them) is far too common. However, good suppliers will always test all their stock in a laboratory; the process is expensive, but it is the only way to find out whether or not an oil is pure. They will also always be willing to give as much information as you need about what you intend to buy – so ask questions about sources, and how the oils are tested and stored.

How long do essential oils last?

Quite simply, the colder the temperature, the longer you can keep your essential oils. The following is a guide to their maximum shelf-life.

- **In the refrigerator**: Once opened, citrus oils (Orange, Lemon, Lime, Mandarin, Tangerine and Bergamot) and Tea Tree will last for one year. All other essential oils will last for two years from opening.

- **At cool room temperature (10°C/55°F)**: Once opened, citrus oils and Tea Tree will last for six months; all other essential oils will last for one year.

Signs to look out for to indicate that your oils are going off are that some go cloudy or sticky in the bottle, some lose the intensity of their fragrance, and some begin to smell sour. If any of these things happen, throw away the oils.

Storing tips

Essential oils are natural substances and they start to go off as soon as you open a bottle because the oil begins to oxidize (see below). To get the most out of your oils follow these guidelines:

• Keep your oils in dark-glass bottles and in a dark place; the UV rays in sunlight make them degrade.

• Keep your oils at a cool temperature (a maximum of 10°C/55°F), as heat makes them go off more quickly. If you keep them in the refrigerator, use a tightly closed box to prevent the oils' aromas from affecting your food.

• Buy oils in screw-cap bottles and keep the caps screwed on tight during storage. The oxygen in the air will degrade the oils if it gets in, a process known as oxidization.

• Once you have opened a bottle of oil for the first time, write the date on a sticky label and place it on the side. Calculate the oil's shelf-life (see opposite) from that date and mark the expiry date on the label. If any oil is left once it reaches that date, feel free to use it as a room fragrance, but do not apply it to your skin or use it in the bath. Old essential oils are more likely to cause allergic skin reactions than fresh ones.

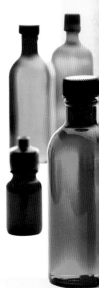

Safety comes first

Essential oils are powerful substances. For example, it takes three-quarters of a tonne of lavender flowers and stalks to produce just 2 litres/66 fl oz of Lavender essential oil, and any extracted essential oil is about 100 times more concentrated than it was in the plant. Smell lavender flowers on a bush and then smell a bottle of the oil – the contrasting intensity will be obvious. To be safe, therefore, we must use essential oils carefully and in small amounts.

Counting the drops

The individual oil profiles given in Part Two of this book provide information on uses and blends for each oil. The safe and effective amounts to use are shown in numbers of drops. (Essential oil bottles have special dropper inserts to dispense one drop at a time, so counting is easy.) It is very important that you never exceed the stated number of drops and that you always read the safety guidelines for every essential oil in every blend.

For the most part, the blends given in Part Two contain even numbers of drops, because there may be times (for example, during pregnancy or for use with children) when you need to make lower concentrations of essential oil blends, and even numbers make it possible to halve the number of drops. However, occasionally, a blend will require only one drop of a certain essential oil, because that oil is particularly pungent or powerful (for example, Black Cumin Seed; pp.192–3). When you need to halve the drops of the other oils in such a blend, it is fine to use one drop of the pungent oil. The blend will smell quite strong, but will still be pleasant thanks to the other oils mixed into it.

Be safe, be wise

It is worth remembering that many essential oils are used today for medicinal purposes, just as they have been used for hundreds of years. None of us would ever take a conventional medicine without first checking its dosage and contraindications to make sure that we are using it safely. Even though essential oils are natural, they must be treated with the same respect. Understanding the safety principles from the start will set you up to enjoy all the benefits that essential oils can bring and to get the best out of aromatherapy, without taking any risks. Therefore, it is important to follow some basic guidelines (see pp.24–9). The following are the two most important safety rules to remember.

- First and most important: **don't ever swallow essential oils.** They are concentrated and highly potent substances, and in large amounts they can attack the delicate linings of the mouth and digestive tract. In sufficiently large doses, swallowing essential oil may cause a poisoning reaction in the body.

- Second: **keep all essential oils well out of the reach of small children.** This is because children have a tendency to put things into their mouths, and as we already know, swallowing essential oils can be dangerous. If you think a small child has swallowed some essential oil, it is always best to seek medical attention straightaway. Take the bottle of oil with you so that the nurse or doctor can advise you appropriately.

23

Skin safety

Whether via an aromatherapy bath or a few drops of a blend rubbed in during massage, the skin is the most usual route by which we enjoy essential oils. The outer layer of our skin has cells that overlap like tiles on a roof, through which the oil is absorbed and eventually enters into the bloodstream.

Avoiding irritation

Irritation is a reaction where an itchy or prickly red rash breaks out suddenly on the skin's surface. To avoid irritation, observe one simple rule: do not use undiluted oils directly on your skin. Always dilute essential oils in blends with a carrier oil (see pp.76–99). However, there are two exceptions: you can use neat Lavender (see pp.134–5) as first aid for burns, cuts and insect bites

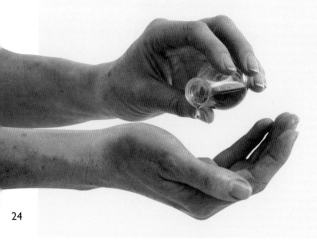

(2 drops on a cotton bud is safe for adults and children); and you can use Tea Tree (pp.138–9) in the same way to treat pimples, cuts, insect bites and warts.

Reducing the risk of sensitization

More serious than irritation, sensitization is an allergic reaction causing swelling and extreme itching on the skin. When selecting an oil from Part Two, read the safety information carefully to see if your choice may cause a reaction. If you do have allergy-prone skin, avoid sensitizing oils altogether, even in blends.

Even if you do not normally have sensitive skin, be aware that allergies can be spontaneous; it's impossible to predict when or if people will react to essential oils – everybody is different. However, using fresh, good-quality oils in low concentrations helps to prevent any allergic reactions.

Dealing with skin reactions

If you have a reaction to an essential oil blend, wash it off with unfragranced soap and apply a plain carrier oil, such as Grapeseed, to calm the area.

Doing a patch test

To test an essential oil on your skin, put 3 drops of the oil in 10ml/2 tsp carrier oil (see pp.76–99) and massage a small amount of this blend into the skin on the inside of your arm. Cover the area with a hypoallergenic plaster (Band Aid) and leave it there overnight. Remove it in the morning – if the skin looks normal, then the oil is safe for you to use.

25

Safety for pregnancy, babies and children

Aromatic back massage is one of the most soothing treatments for a pregnant woman, especially when nearing labour; scented baby massage is wonderful to relax a baby and reinforce the parental bond; and small children often enjoy smelling gentle essential oils to soothe away stress or anxiety. However, in all these scenarios it is crucial to use the right oils in the correct amounts.

Safety during pregnancy

- Do not use any massage blends with essential oils or any oils in your baths until *after* your first three months of pregnancy.
- Massage blends in pregnancy should contain half the numbers of drops of essential oils in any normal blend. For example, if a normal blend contains 4 drops Roman Chamomile and 2 drops Lavender in 20ml/4 tsp carrier oil, for pregnancy reduce this to 2 drops Roman Chamomile and 1 drop Lavender in the same amount of carrier oil.

Avoid: The following oils have strong purifying effects, so are too intense for pregnancy – Rosemary (p.112), Spanish Sage (p.114), Yarrow (p.122), Myrrh (p.150), Laurel Leaf (p.156), Fennel (p.200), Juniper Berry (p.202), Agnus Castus (p.210), Sweet Basil (p.218), Tulsi (Indian Holy Basil; p.220), Damiana (p.222), Angelica Root (p.226), Lovage Root (p.242), Jasmine Absolute (p.260).

Special recommendations: The following oils are all soothing and relaxing, so are ideal for massage after the first three months of pregnancy – Roman Chamomile (p.124), Orange Leaf (p.130), Lavender (p.134), Geranium (p.142),

Lemon (p.182), Australian Sandalwood (p.208), Sweet Orange (p.232), Neroli (p.256), Mandarin (p.258), Rose Otto (p.268).

Safety for babies and toddlers

Never use essential oils on babies younger than three months old. Once a baby has reached the three-month stage, you can use 1 drop of just one essential oil diluted in 20ml/4 tsp carrier oil per massage application or baby bath. For example, for a baby massage you could use 1 drop Rose Otto in 20ml/4 tsp Sweet Almond oil. Only the following four oils are safe for babies and toddlers: Roman Chamomile (p.124; to heal a sore bottom), Lavender (p.134; to aid sleep and soothe the skin), Neroli (p.256; to calm fretfulness) and Rose Otto (p.268; to moisturize the skin).

Safety for two- to ten-year-olds

Never combine more than 2 drops each of two essential oils in a massage blend intended for children aged between two and ten years old. That is, you should never have more than 4 drops in total in 20ml/4 tsp carrier oil. Children over the age of ten can be treated using standard adult blends.

Heavily scented oils tend not to appeal to children, so the following is a selection of safe, gently aromatic and useful oils: Roman Chamomile (p.124; to soothe the nerves), Lavender (p.134; to aid sleep), Lemon-scented Eucalyptus (p.152; to relieve colds), Lemon (p.182; to unblock the nose), Sweet Orange (p.232; to calm emotional stress), Spearmint (p.248; to relieve tummy aches), Neroli (p.256; to aid sleep) and Rose Otto (p.268; to soothe skin irritation). **27**

Safety in the sun

If you like to get out in the sun at the first sign of summer, or if you take regular trips to the local sunbed parlour, you need to be careful about which essential oils you apply to your skin. Some oils – mainly from the peel of certain citrus fruits, although there are one or two others – contain biochemical ingredients that can cause a skin reaction under exposure to the UV rays of strong sunlight, or sunbeds. These oils are known as "phototoxic", and the reaction on your skin is "photosensitivity", which causes irregular patches of dark tanning, or, in severe cases, actual burns. Photosensitivity is an issue only when you apply phototoxic oils to your skin via massage blends. It does not apply when you use these oils in the bath or in a shower-gel (because you wash them off), nor does it apply to vaporizers and inhalations.

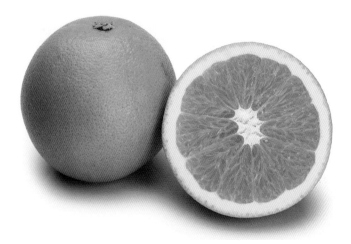

Sun-safe citrus oils

Although most citrus essential oils *are* phototoxic (see below), modern perfumery research has shown that those of Sweet Orange, Tangerine and Mandarin are *not*, and that you can apply them to skin exposed to UV rays with no problems. However, check the safety information in Part Two for any oil that you intend to use on exposed areas of skin before you apply it.

Phototoxic essential oils

All the oils profiled in Part Two are safe to use on areas of skin that are exposed to sunlight or the UV rays of a sunbed, except for the following:

- Bergamot (p.132)
- Lemon (p.182)
- Angelica Root (p.226)
- Grapefruit (p.228)
- Lovage Root (p.242)
- Lime (p.254)

If you do want to use any of these oils in the summer or alongside your usual sunbed routine, apply them diluted in massage blends (with a carrier oil) as normal, but then leave a minimum of 12 hours before exposing your skin to UV rays, to give your body time to process the oils.

How we absorb essential oils

The chemical make-up of essential oils is extremely complex. Most oils contain an average of 150 biochemical constituents, and some – such as Rose Otto – are made up of more than 300. It is these constituents that work individually and synergistically to have positive effects on our mind, body and spirit. And it is their tiny molecules that make it easy for the oils to penetrate the human body in two main ways – by slipping through the skin and by being breathed in from the air.

Slipping through the skin

The skin provides a large surface area, the top layer of which comprises overlapping cells that, during massage or in an aromatherapy bath, allow the small essential-oil molecules to pass through and into the bloodstream. Once in the bloodstream, essential oils will bring about their specific effects (for example, help the immune system to fight bacteria, soothe aching muscles or potentially increase endorphin levels) and will then be processed by the kidneys, to be passed out of the system some 12 hours later in the urine.

We can enhance the process of absorbing essential oils if we apply them to the skin using rubbing, stroking or massaging movements. Rubbing the oils into your body, in whichever way feels comfortable for you, expands tiny capillaries below the skin's surface. This increases blood-flow to the area, enabling the essential oils to be absorbed rapidly into your muscle tissue. You are likely to feel the physical effects of the oils as warmth or tingling sensations – signs that tension and stiffness are beginning to ease away and that the many other benefits of the oils are just around the corner.

However, massage is not the only way in which we can encourage essential oils to be absorbed through the skin. Taking a warm bath plumps up and softens the normally hard surface cells of the skin, making them more permeable. This allows essential oils to penetrate the skin's upper layers, just as they do in massage. So, by placing essential oils in our bathwater, we can turn an ordinary bath into an aromatherapy treatment. Aromatherapy baths are particularly gentle, because a few drops of essential oil are spread out widely over a relatively large volume of water. In this way, the skin absorbs the essential oils in much smaller amounts than during massage.

Breathed in from the air

While some drops of essential oil float on the water's surface in a warm bath so that we can absorb them through our skin, others will respond to the heat in the bathwater and rise into the air as fragrant steam. When we breathe in this steam, the tiny molecules that make up essential oils reach the air passages inside the nose, as well as the deeper passages of the respiratory system, so that we can literally breathe in their benefits.

We can concentrate this effect by using pungent, cleansing essential oils (such as Eucalyptus) in inhalation treatments (see pp.56–7) to clear blocked sinuses, a blocked nose, or congestion in the throat and chest when we have a bad cold or cough. Furthermore, some essential oils (such as Tea Tree) have antimicrobial effects in the air as well as in the body, so that, even before we breathe them in, they set to work killing airborne germs and protecting us from further infection, or from spreading our infection to others.

31

The science of essential oils

Only around 10 per cent of the total annual world output of essential oils is used in aromatherapy – the rest is divided between the pharmaceutical, food and fragrance industries. These industries have supported essential-oil research to establish what is safe to put on the skin and what is safe to consume (minute amounts of essential oils may be used as natural flavourings). Along the way, scientists have made several key discoveries about the healing properties of essential oils. Here are some of them.

Fighting viruses

Our immune system alone must deal with fighting a virus such as flu, because antibiotics can't help. US research suggests that essential oils such as Melissa (p.262) may stop viruses replicating, so that the immune system can overcome them more easily.

Avoiding fungal infections

Research in Australia and India has shown that Lemongrass (p.104), Tea Tree (p.138) and Coriander Seed (p.234) are effective against several fungal infections, such as athlete's foot (use 4–6 drops in a foot bath a third full with warm water) and candidiasis (put 4–6 drops in your bathwater).

Lowering blood pressure

High blood pressure is often characterized by constricted (narrowed) arteries, which need to open to allow blood to flow more freely. Opening up the arteries is called vasodilation, and scientists in the UK have found that both

Lavender (p.134) and Geranium (p.142) essential oils are good vasodilators. This means that these oils are "hypotensive" – they lower blood pressure. (If you suffer from high blood pressure, talk to your doctor before you begin any complementary treatment, in case it interferes with your medication.)

Coping with epilepsy

In therapeutic trials with epileptic subjects, inhaling strongly camphor-rich essential oils, such as Spike Lavender (p.108), Rosemary (p.112) or Yarrow (p.122) has been shown to slightly increase seizure rates. Relaxing essential oils, such as Lavender (p.134) and Ylang Ylang (p.250), have been shown to reduce seizure rates and even help to prevent seizures altogether. However, if you suffer from epilepsy, talk to your doctor before using any essential oils.

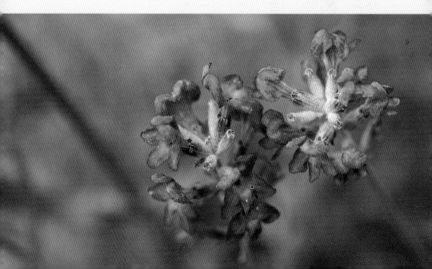

The power of scent

Our amazing sense of smell is more than just a physical function: it can transport us to a memory of another place or time, and even to another mood. Through it we can interpret many thousands of aromas, often in an instant; it affects us all the time and yet somehow we hardly ever notice it.

Cross-section showing the olfactory pathways of the left nostril

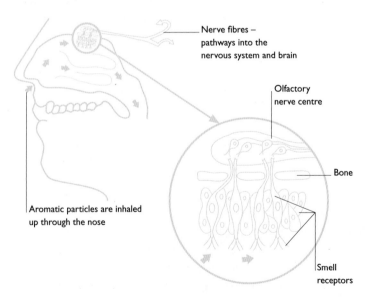

Nerve fibres – pathways into the nervous system and brain

Olfactory nerve centre

Bone

Aromatic particles are inhaled up through the nose

Smell receptors

How the sense of smell works

When we breathe in, air carrying thousands of aromatic particles is drawn up the nostrils. At the back of the nasal cavity is the olfactory nerve centre where two patches of tiny cells, the "smell receptors", link to the nervous system (see diagram, left). These cells trap the aromatic molecules and then send out tiny impulses into and along nerve fibres, which end in the centre of the brain where we interpret smell. This whole process takes under two seconds. Once the brain has received repeated impulses of the same smell, it "switches off" its response, which is why we stop noticing a smell after a while.

Smell responses

There are two main types of response to an aroma. The first type involves instinctive or automatic gestures, such as opening your eyes wide in pleasure or turning away your head in disgust. It also includes making appreciative or unappreciative noises about smells – sounds such as "mmm" or "ughh". These kinds of response are linked to areas of instinctive behaviour deep inside the brain, as well as to memories that we may no longer consciously recall (such as those of early childhood), so that they *seem* instinctive. The second type of response occurs when the olfactory impulse travels to the upper levels of the brain, where we store conscious memories. In this case our response is likely to be more verbal and analytical. We might say such things as, "That smell reminds me of ...". Children tend to have the instinctive kind of response to a smell, while adults are likely to have either response, or both responses combined – usually the non-verbal first and the more analytical next.

Aroma, mood and behaviour

Human beings have used aromas for their positive effects on the mind and emotions for millennia. In the eighth century CE, the Chinese philosopher Wang Wei said, "Look into the perfumes of flowers and of Nature for peace of mind and joy of life." In Ancient Egypt, a special perfume recipe, *kyphi*, was said to relieve anxiety, brighten dreams and heal the soul. These are the precursors to one of modern aromatherapy's main aims – to improve mood.

Influencing mood

We often take our sense of smell for granted, only really recognizing its value when it's not there – for example, when we have a blocked nose, causing our food to taste bland and the outside world to seem distant. Once our sense of smell returns, we regain our appetite and we feel more positive and energized again. In short, our sense of smell, or lack of it, directly affects how we feel.

With this in mind, we can use aromas to encourage different kinds of mood. Floral essential oils, such as Rose Absolute or Rose Otto (pp.266 and 268), are uplifting; citrus oils, such as Grapefruit (p.228), are fresh and ease depression; woody oils, such as Australian Sandalwood (p.208), are calming; oils with musky aromas, such as Jasmine Absolute (p.260), are sensual; and studies investigating vaporized Lavender essential oil (p.134), as a sleep-enhancer have shown that the aroma has significant calming mental effects. Furthermore, all essential-oil aromas reconnect us with Nature and an inherent state of relaxation that can simultaneously balance and uplift our mood. The effects are even more enhanced when oils are blended to suit individual smell preferences, as the more you like a fragrance, the better you will feel!

Aromachology – smells and behaviour

If you ask a real estate agent what you can do to help to sell your house, he or she will almost certainly mention that you should brew some fresh coffee just before a potential buyer arrives; even better, bake a cake! These comforting smells help people to feel good in your home, making it seem like a place where they could live. Is this just agent spin? Apparently not. Scientists in the US are doing considerable research into ways that aromas can directly affect human behaviour, particularly when it comes to shopping. One test showed that the right kinds of aroma in a store can genuinely influence what people buy. For example, synthetic bakery smells seem to make people buy more bread – even if the bread is baked off-site!

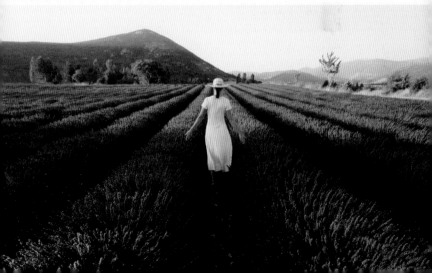

Carrier oils

As we have seen, most essential oils must be diluted in a carrier oil before we can apply them to the skin in massage (see pp.24–5). However, carrier oils do far more than simply act as diluting agents. They are natural vegetable oils that even on their own give wonderful nourishment to the skin. Made up of chains of different fatty acids (see p.276), as well as vitamins and minerals, carrier oils – whether used alone or with essential oils in massage – are absorbed by the upper layers of the skin, leaving a soft, silky finish.

Natural versus synthetic

Although in theory you could use baby oil (or any fatty oil) as a carrier, this is not ideal for aromatherapy. Baby oil is a mineral oil, a synthetic petroleum by-product that merely acts as a slippery barrier over the skin. Natural vegetable oils, on the other hand, are readily absorbed by the skin because they have smaller molecules, making them closer to the skin's own natural oil (sebum).

Basic carriers (pp.76–83)
These oils include Apricot Kernel, Grapeseed, Sunflower and Sweet Almond (all featured in Part Two). Use them for full-body aromatherapy massage treatments, as they provide good skin lubrication so that massage movements flow easily; they also absorb well into the skin.

Skin foods (pp.84–99)
These specialist carrier oils have particular skin-nourishing properties and care for the skin at a deep level, helping cell regeneration. Skin foods are

sometimes added to basic carriers to enrich them, especially when the recipient suffers from dry skin. They also nourish the face, replenishing skin that has been affected by wind or sun, or healing blemishes or broken veins. Included in this group are Aloe Vera extract, used as a gel, for its soothing properties, as well as the oils of Avocado, Borage Seed, Camellia, Evening Primrose, Jojoba, Kukui Nut and Macadamia Nut.

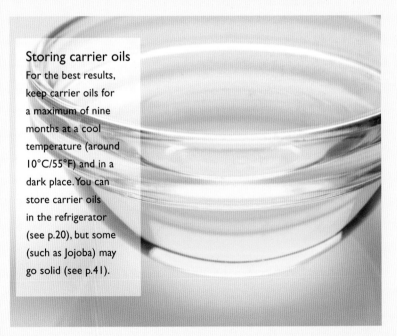

Storing carrier oils

For the best results, keep carrier oils for a maximum of nine months at a cool temperature (around 10°C/55°F) and in a dark place. You can store carrier oils in the refrigerator (see p.20), but some (such as Jojoba) may go solid (see p.41).

39

Aromatherapy blends

An aromatherapy blend is a combination of a carrier oil and one or more essential oils. Shaking together a few drops of essential oil in a carrier (or two carriers if you are enriching your massage base with a skin food; see pp.84–99) makes the essential oil safe to apply to your skin. In professional aromatherapy training, making blends is one of the core skills – it is the aromatherapist's art. A practitioner must not only know which oils contain which healing properties and be able to select them appropriately, he or she also needs to know how the scents of the chosen essential oils will work together to produce something that is both therapeutic *and* smells lovely.

Every oil entry in Part Two includes several suggested blends, each for a specific purpose. All these blends have been carefully chosen for maximum effectiveness and safety, based on my 16 years of aromatherapy practice. If you want to experiment with blending, it's a good idea to take a course in aromatherapy to learn in depth about essential oils.

Making a blend

Before you make your blend, make sure that you have a clean, dark-glass bottle in which to mix it. The dark glass will prevent the blend from spoiling as a result of the UV rays in sunlight (see p.21). Essential-oil suppliers and most good pharmacies will sell bottles in 20ml/4 tsp or 50ml/10 tsp sizes; for the blends in this book, the smaller size should be enough. Measure in 20ml/4 tsp of your chosen carrier oil. Then, add the drops of essential oils listed in the formula you have selected. Screw the lid on the bottle and shake. The blend is now ready to use.

All the blends in this book are calculated for 20ml/4 tsp carrier oil. This is enough blended oil for one full-body massage, or for several applications to your arms or legs. Blends will last between four and six weeks if you keep them at room temperature (around 15°C/60°F). Or you can keep most blends for up to three months in the refrigerator, but be aware that some carriers (such as Jojoba) will go solid. If this does happen, simply remove the blend from the refrigerator and allow it to liquefy again at room temperature.

Blend dilutions

I have calculated most of the blends in Part Two as a total of 10 drops in 20ml/4 tsp carrier oil. This is the most commonly used dilution for massage on normal adult skin. People with sensitive skin and pregnant women past the first trimester should use only *half* the number of drops in 20ml/4 tsp carrier oil. This is a safe, lower concentration. If you are pregnant or suffer from sensitive skin, look out for the less-concentrated, gentle blends in Part Two. Note that some of the pregnancy blends are suitable only for women who have passed their second trimester (six months) – these are clearly marked.

A blend of three

In Part Two you will see that most of the massage blends I've suggested contain three essential oils. This creates a well-balanced, pleasing fragrance, in the same way that the top, middle and base notes work in perfumery (see p.276).

Making a skin mousse

If your skin is extremely dry or sensitive, or if it is in any way sun-damaged, a standard blend of essential oil in a carrier oil will not soothe redness, irritation or burns. Instead, you will need a special alternative to deeply nourish and repair your skin, which is why I have created my very own Skin Mousse formula. Easy to make and to apply, it is made up of pure-quality Aloe Vera gel (see pp.86–7), to cool and hydrate the skin and reduce inflammation, combined with Jojoba carrier oil (see pp.98–9), a liquid wax that is similar to the skin's own natural oils and has superb softening properties. The Skin Mousse works wonderfully as a special face treatment, to apply to problem areas of skin anywhere on the body, or as a soft, soothing treat for baby skin.

Making the mousse

Take a clean glass jar that is big enough to hold up to 20ml/4 tsp of the finished mousse. Add 15ml/3 flat tsp Aloe Vera gel, then 5ml/1 tsp Jojoba carrier oil and stir the mixture with a small spoon. The oil and gel will start to combine and thicken. At this point, add another 2.5ml/½ tsp Aloe Vera gel and keep stirring. The mixture will suddenly go smooth and slack, taking on an opaque, pale cream colour. You will have approximately 20ml/4 tsp mousse in total – enough for around ten applications to the face.

You can use the mousse unfraganced, or, if you prefer, you can try one of the mousse blends suggested in Part Two (see p.103 for an example), by adding the relevant essential oils in the stated amounts, and stirring again. The mousse will last between four and six weeks at a cool room temperature (around 10°C/55°F) and will leave your skin feeling calmed, restored and soft.

My own "Eureka!" moment

I created this Skin Mousse for myself when I had a bad outbreak of hives on my neck and chest. The itching was almost unbearable, and one night, at three in the morning, I was sitting in my kitchen thinking, "What can I do?" Then, as if by magic, the formula jumped into my head. I was surprised because I had never thought to combine Aloe Vera gel and Jojoba before, but it worked like a treat, even without essential oils. I simply put it unfragranced on my skin and it soothed the angry patches straightaway. I have added many combinations of essential oils to it since, with great results for all kinds of skin problems.

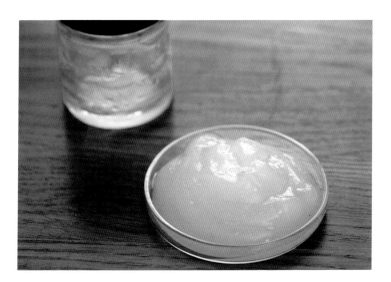

Using essential oils

People often ask me whether it's possible to use essential oils too much, or whether it's possible to overdose on them. These are sensible questions because, as we have already seen, essential oils are highly concentrated substances with powerful effects.

What and how often?

If you want to enjoy essential oils in your daily life, adding them to baths is a great way to start. Try taking an evening aromatherapy bath (see pp.54–5). Soak in it for 20 minutes or so, towel yourself dry, and then rub in a blend. If you need to unwind after a hard day, a bath blend such as 4 drops Frankincense, 2 drops Rose Otto and 4 drops Neroli will calm your mind, and also help to replenish your skin (see p.127). Informal massage (simply rubbing the oils into the skin) is another good starting point. If you stick to the guidelines on the following pages and make up blends as directed in Part Two, you will be using only tiny amounts of oils in low concentrations, which are easy for your body to process. These applications are suitable for daily use.

Integrating other methods of application into your daily routine is helpful when you need to treat a particular issue. For example, if you have a cold, you could do an inhalation (see pp.56–7) to clear your head and nose two or three times a day; and you could use a vaporizer (see pp.58–9) to kill the airborne germs, also two or three times a day. A bath with antimicrobial essential oils, such as Tea Tree or Manuka, will also help the body to fight the

The blends in this book are wonderful for daily massage – whether to treat specific problems such as abdominal pain or aching limbs, or simply to uplift your mood and restore vitality.

virus. During illnesses such as colds and flu, using several methods is extremely beneficial as it gets the oils into the system in various ways, easing away the different symptoms of illness and boosting immunity from different angles.

Can you use too much?

The only way in which you could ever really use too much essential oil is if you swallowed it, which the safety guidelines (see pp.22–3) indicate that you should *never* do. So, as long as you never drink any essential oil, it is unlikely that you will ever manage to overdose. Regularly using low concentrations of essential oils safely is nothing but beneficial to your health and well-being.

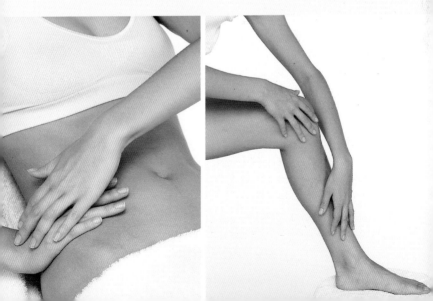

Benefits and applications

Aromatherapy has so many benefits. Some are obvious, such as recovering from a cold or relieving the pain of a pulled muscle. Others are more subtle and instinctive responses to aromas, such as feeling emotional tension dissolve or getting a wonderful night's sleep. Aromatherapy enables us to discover more about our senses – particularly touch and smell – and the subtle changes that our senses can create in our mind and mood. Even those who are not able to communicate verbally can feel these benefits. For example, a client of mine who is severely affected by dementia always relaxes immediately when I vaporize Lavender in her room. The more you experience essential oils, the more their benefits will filter into your consciousness.

Getting the best out of essential oils means choosing the most suitable way to use them for you, depending upon your treatment needs and preferences. Sometimes two or three methods work well together. For example, if you are stressed at work and it is keeping you awake at night, an evening aromatherapy bath and then a self-massage with relaxing essential oils will help you to sleep. You can also try using a vaporizer (see pp.58–9) on your desk with refreshing essential oils to help you to concentrate.

You will find out on pages 48–61 how to apply and use essential oils. Each method has particular benefits, which are summarized below to help you to select the best approach to suit your needs at any given time.

• **Massage:** Smooth, long massage strokes have been scientifically proven to reduce blood pressure and ease stress. More vigorous massage improves the circulation, eases out muscular spasm and soothes aches and pains.

Massaging in a blend made up of quality carrier oil and a combination of specific essential oils helps to nourish your skin. You can find out more about how to perform aromatherapy massage on pages 48–53.

- **Baths:** Deeply relaxing, aromatherapy baths are especially recommended at night to switch off the mind and prepare you for sleep. By adding particular essential oils to the water, you can help to ease problems such as stress or anxiety (see Part Two for specific recommendations). You can find out more about how to prepare an aromatherapy bath and some ideal blends to use on pages 54–5.

- **Inhalations:** An inhalation is highly beneficial if you have flu, a cold, sinusitis or hay fever, as it will help to unblock your respiratory passages and ease your breathing. Find out more about inhalations on pages 56–7.

- **Vaporizers:** A vaporizer releases the aroma of essential oils into a room. You may use one simply to create a pleasant atmosphere or, more specifically, to ease symptoms of respiratory troubles, to aid concentration or to envelop yourself in calm. Find out more about vaporizers on pages 58–9.

- **Compresses:** If you have a minor injury, such as a sprain or strain, a compress will provide the perfect first-aid treatment; and compresses containing a cleansing essential oil such as Yarrow (see pp.122–3) can help to disinfect wounds. Find out more about compresses on pages 60–61.

Preparing to give massage

Whether you plan to massage yourself or a partner, preparation is key. Start by setting up the right kind of space for your massage (see below) and be sure to have all your materials to hand – including any aromatherapy blends (already blended) that you intend to use. Also bear in mind that massage is not always appropriate – there are circumstances in which it wouldn't be safe to have or give a massage. Before you begin, check the chart opposite and, if any of the symptoms apply, either avoid massage altogether or make the necessary modifications. In addition, note that while massage with a loved one can be sensual and fun, you should avoid using essential oils (including in blends) in erotic massage, as they can cause condoms to degenerate.

Creating a massage space

A clean, uncluttered environment will enhance any massage treatment. If you are giving someone else a massage, ask them to lie on the floor on a large pad, such as a futon mattress or large floor cushion. Cover the pad with clean bath towels, and have more clean towels to hand so that you can cover your partner's body with them after you have treated specific areas. Make sure that there are plenty of cushions to support his or her head and knees. The room should be warm; even so, a blanket over the legs will stop your partner feeling cold – remove and replace it according to which areas you are massaging. Have some paper towels ready to mop up any oil spills. Don't start the treatment until you have released your own stress: centre yourself for a few moments – then start. Whether you are massaging someone else or yourself, switch off your phone and play some peaceful music to help to set the mood.

Contraindications to massage

Run through this checklist before you massage yourself or a partner.

SYMPTOM	ACTION
• High temperature/colds/flu	• Avoid massage. The body is fighting infection and needs rest.
• Headache/migraine	• A professional massage therapist may use specific techniques to help; beginners should avoid massage.
• Varicose veins	• Experienced therapists work above and below the affected areas, but beginners should avoid massage.
• Inflammation (for example, as a result of an injury)	• Avoid massage, as the practice could worsen the condition.
• Physical injury (for example, a broken bone)	• Avoid massage, which could increase any pain and swelling.
• Pregnancy	• Massage is suitable only after the first trimester (three months), and then only gentle, soothing strokes.

49

Massage strokes

Massage is much more effective if you learn and use some specific massage techniques. The strokes that follow are simple to apply and can be used anywhere on the body, from the back, neck and shoulders to the legs and feet. Quicker-paced strokes are invigorating, while slower strokes are more relaxing. They will all work in self-massage, too.

- **Effleurage (1):** This French word means "stroking". With the entire palms of the hands, apply long, flowing movements along the body, for example applying pressure from the lower back up toward the shoulders, then easing the hands down again. Use this stroke at the start of a massage as it warms the skin, eases out the muscles and helps the body and mind to relax into the treatment.

- **Knuckling (2):** This stroke is slightly more stimulating than effleurage. Loosely clench your fists and, pressing gently with the knuckles, work over fleshy areas such as the outsides of the thighs and the tops of the shoulders. Knuckling eases out tension in the muscles and improves blood supply, making the muscles feel invigorated and refreshed.

- **Kneading "double-handed" (3):** If you have ever made bread, this double-handed stroke is like wringing out dough! It is best used on the side of the abdomen, on the sides of the back or over the shoulders. Pick up the flesh and squeeze it between the thumb and forefingers of one hand, then the other, in a rhythmical movement. This stroke works tension out of muscles.

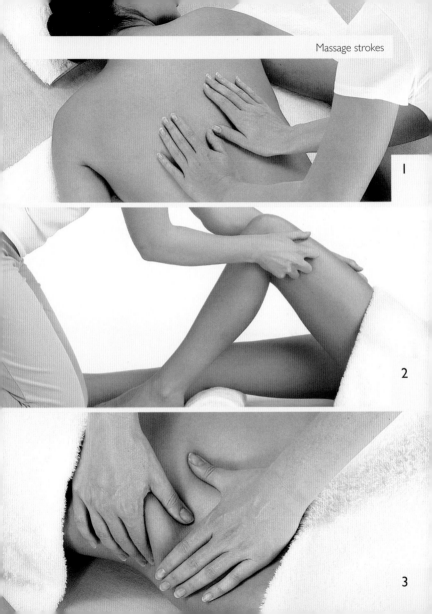

1

2

3

More massage strokes

This second selection of massage strokes will add variety and depth to your massage routines, easing tension in different parts of the body.

• **Fanning (1):** This variation of effleurage (see p.50) is a warming massage stroke and works well on the back, as it is good for relaxing large areas of muscle tissue. Place your hands on either side of the base of your partner's spine. Press down and fan your hands out toward the sides of the body. Slowly move your hands up slightly and repeat the technique. Four or five fanning movements are usually enough to cover the back from the base of the spine to the shoulders. In self-massage, this technique can ease out muscular tension in the tops of the thighs.

• **Thumb pressures (2):** This technique works well in the natural grooves on either side of the spine. Place one thumb on each side of the base of your partner's spine, about 2.5cm/1 in apart. Lean into the thumbs to apply pressure for a few seconds, then ease off. Check with your partner that the pressure is comfortable. Move the thumbs up about 2.5cm/1 in and repeat. Do this all the way up the back. In self-massage, thumb pressures work well in lines from the knee, up across the top of the thigh and out toward the outside of the hip, to overcome cellulite.

• **Reflex stroke (3):** This relaxing stroke is good to end a treatment. Glide your hands gently over the massaged area, one after the other, in a flowing movement. Make your touch gradually lighter as you finish the massage.

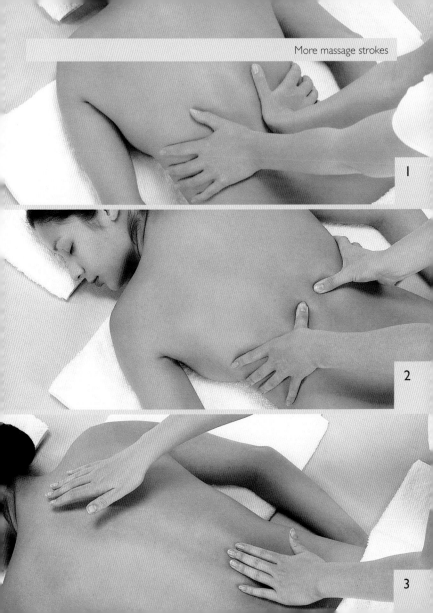

Aromatherapy baths

If you need to switch off from your day and you want some "time out", take a bath; even better, take an aromatherapy bath – one that is enhanced with essential oils. An aromatherapy bath is a form of holistic treatment, partly because you relax in the warm water, but specifically because of the fragrant effects of the oils you add. As well as finding their way into your body by gently lapping at your skin, the oils vaporize in the steam of the warm bathwater, meaning that you inhale their benefits, too. As refreshing as it can be to take a shower with an essential-oil-enhanced shower gel, sadly it won't do the same job – only an aromatherapy bath will truly ease your mind.

Preparing an essential-oil bath

Light some candles around the bathroom and play some soft music to create a relaxing atmosphere. Run the water to a comfortable temperature. Once the bath is run, swirl in *one* of the following water-softening ingredients, depending on the kind of treatment you want.

• To detoxify all the body's systems: 120g/4oz Epsom salts
• To soften the water and soothe the skin: 120ml/4 fl oz full-cream milk
• To nourish dry skin: 10ml/2 tsp unfragranced dispersing bath oil (available from essential-oil suppliers)

Then add your chosen essential oils (see box, opposite, for some suggestions) – up to a total of 6 drops. Finally, get into the water and soak for at least 20 minutes (top up the bath with hot water if necessary). Relax and enjoy.

54

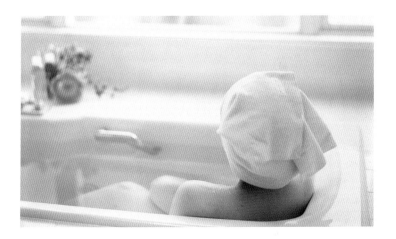

Bath combinations to relax and restore

The following bath blends are suitable for all adults, unless you have sensitive skin or are pregnant. If you do have sensitive skin or are pregnant (and past your first trimester), you should halve the drops in each of these combinations.

- To relax: 2 drops Ylang Ylang and 4 drops Sweet Orange
- To improve sleep: 4 drops Lavender and 2 drops Australian Sandalwood
- To detoxify the body's systems: 2 drops Myrtle and 4 drops Grapefruit
- To soothe the skin: 2 drops Roman Chamomile and 4 drops Geranium

Aromatherapy inhalations

An aromatherapy inhalation is a few drops of essential oil added to hot water to create a therapeutic steam. Inhaling this steam can help to open your airways and improve your breathing, especially during colds, flu, hay fever and sinusitis. The essential oil travels in the vapour up your nose, where its tiny molecules help to loosen blockages and soothe any swollen mucous membranes in the nasal passages. As your breath deepens, essential-oil vapour also travels down the main respiratory passages toward the lungs, easing coughs and tight chests. It is best to use an inhalation first thing in the morning and last thing in the evening when your cold symptoms will tend to feel worse, with an extra inhalation at midday if you need it.

How to do an inhalation

Half-fill a large heatproof bowl with near-boiling water. If you wear spectacles or contact lenses, remove them. Add to the water up to 6 drops, in total, of essential oils (see box, right), then lean over the fragrant steam with a towel draped over your head and the bowl. Lift the towel from time to time to let in some cool air so that you don't begin to feel uncomfortable. Breathe slowly, deeply and steadily, allowing the aromatic vapour to enter your nose and lungs, for up to 15 minutes. You will feel the penetrating vapours of the essential oils clearing your head and nose, bringing lightness and relief.

Safety note: If you are an asthma-sufferer, you should avoid inhalations as the combination of steam and essential oils may be too intense for you. Instead, take an aromatherapy bath (see pp.54–5) to help to ease your breathing.

Inhalation combinations to clear and soothe

The following inhalation blends are suitable for all adults, except those who suffer from asthma (see safety note, opposite).

- To ease a stuffy head: 3 drops Eucalyptus and 3 drops Scots Pine
- To unblock the nose: 3 drops Myrtle and 3 drops Peppermint
- To soothe the throat and chest: 3 drops Himalayan Cedarwood and 3 drops Frankincense
- To help to ease a chest infection: 3 drops Tea Tree and 3 drops Lemon

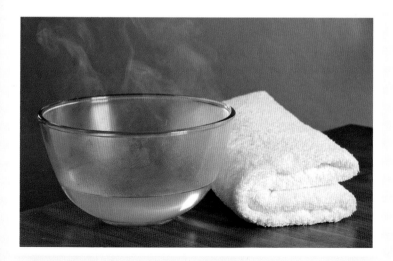

Using a vaporizer

Vaporizing an essential oil (heating it up to release the aromatic molecules into the air) can achieve many things. First, it can create a special atmosphere in a room for a particular task or event. For example, calming Frankincense prepares a space for meditation; while an uplifting oil, such as Orange or Lemon (3 drops of each, individually or combined), can prepare a welcoming space for a dinner party (uplifting aromas help people to feel at ease; see opposite for some ideas). Second, and more practically, if someone in the house has a cold or flu, regularly using vaporizers with antimicrobial essential oils, such as Tea Tree (see pp.138–9), helps to eliminate germs from the air and to prevent other household members from catching the infection. Finally, research has shown that using Lavender essential oil in vaporizers as we go to bed is a natural and gentle way to improve our quality of sleep.

Finding the right equipment

Most pharmacies and oil suppliers will sell electric vaporizers that gently heat or fan essential oils so that their molecules float into the air. You can leave electric models working all night, so they are particularly useful if you intend to use oils to help with sleep or breathing problems. Some types of electric vaporizer have a pad in the base to which you add the essential oils and a fan that spreads the aroma; while others (such as those shown opposite) plug in and heat up so that the essential oil evaporates from the vaporizer's surface. Traditional essential-oil burners have a candle beneath a glass or ceramic "tray" into which you drop the oils. These work well, but for fire-safety reasons may be best avoided, especially if you have children or are elderly.

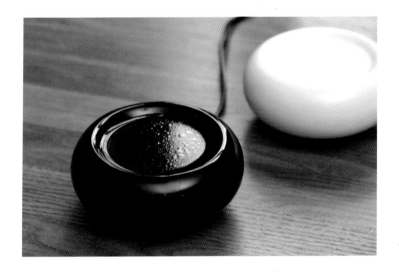

Vaporizer combinations to improve mood and well-being

Placing one of the following combinations in a traditional vaporizer with a tray or in an electric one (shown above) will scent a room for about one hour.

- To make a room feel relaxing: 2 drops Lemongrass and 4 drops Cardamom
- To warm guests and lift the spirits at a winter gathering: 4 drops Sweet Orange and 2 drops Clove Bud
- To keep germs at bay: 3 drops Tea Tree and 3 drops Manuka
- To improve sleep: 4 drops Lavender and 2 drops Tangerine

Using a compress

Cold and hot compresses (a few drops of essential oil placed on a cold or warm damp cloth) provide essential-oil first aid – use them to treat minor injuries, such as sprains, muscle strains, cuts and grazes. You will need a piece of cloth, preferably a muslin square or a clean dish towel, as well as a medium-sized bowl filled with cold or hot water, according to which type of compress you want to use. Then, you simply place not more than 6 drops, in total, of your chosen essential oils on the surface of the water and soak them up into the cloth (see below). All the combinations I have suggested here are suitable for anyone to use, including children and pregnant women.

Cold compresses

Use a cold compress to treat injuries such as a sprained ankle or a pulled muscle. Add the oil drops to the surface of the water and then lay your cloth over the water to absorb the drops, without dipping it in. This will be enough to "collect" the drops of oil and dilute them slightly. Try adding ice to the bowl to make the water really cold, as this will help to reduce any inflammation and soothe away any pain. Gently wring out the cloth, and then apply it to the injured area. Keep the injury raised and leave the compress in place for 20 minutes. If your injury is acute, repeat the process twice more straightaway and seek medical help. The box, opposite, suggests blends for a cold compress.

Hot compresses

Use a hot compress to draw out infection from cuts and wounds. The water in the bowl should be hot, but bearable to touch. Place the drops of essential

Effective combinations for cold compresses

Good essential-oil combinations to use in a cold compress are:

- To relieve muscular pain: 3 drops German Chamomile and 3 drops Lavender
- To cool and calm inflammation: 3 drops Peppermint and 3 drops Yarrow
- To ease a pulled muscle: 3 drops Roman Chamomile and 3 drops Sweet Marjoram

Effective combinations for hot compresses

Good essential-oil combinations to use in a hot compress are:

- For scratches and grazes: 3 drops Tea Tree and 3 drops Frankincense
- For deep, infected cuts: 3 drops Myrrh and 3 drops Manuka
- For boils or infected pimples: 3 drops Bergamot and 3 drops Ravensara

oil onto the surface of the water and then lay over the piece of cloth, as advised for the cold compress. Remove the cloth immediately and gently wring it out. Apply the compress to the wound for approximately 20 minutes, and then either throw away the cloth and use a brand new one next time, or sterilize it by boiling it in water for 20 minutes. You will need to repeat the process two or three times in a row to draw out the infection. See the box above for good blends to use with a hot compress.

Grouping the oils together

The oils in Part Two are grouped together in two main ways. First, there are the carrier oils, which are themselves grouped into basic carriers and "skin foods" (those carriers that are particularly soothing to the skin). Second, there are the essential oils, which are grouped according to their most potent health-giving properties (see below). We all have different smell preferences, so having a range of oils to choose from in any group means that there is bound to be something for everyone. By linking each group to both physical and emotional issues, I hope to allow you to get the most out of essential oils – to choose them wisely and precisely – and to encourage you to experiment with oils to test their effects on your own spirit and sense of well-being.

Understanding the groups of essential oils

The groups I have chosen – Muscle Treats, Skin Enhancers, Easy Breathers, Warming Stimulants, Immune Boosters, Hormone Harmonizers, Nerve Relievers, Digestive Soothers and Uplifting Aromas – not only represent aromatherapy's most successful applications, they are also the main reasons why clients tend to come for aromatherapy treatments. However, even though a particular oil is grouped under a main function, this is by no means its only function, so many of the oils appear in blends in other groupings, too.

Choosing the best oils for you

If you have a particular problem or ailment, use the Contents page or Index to find the section that is linked to the group of oils you need. Read through the profiles of the oils in that grouping, and see which oils seem to link closely to your issue. If possible, take the book along to your local supplier and smell the essential oils in that group – your nose and brain are very clever and through them you will know instinctively which oils are best for you. Remember that the therapeutic benefits of an essential oil are to do with how much you enjoy its scent, as well as its physical healing properties. So, if, when you smell a particular essential oil, your mind clears, and you smile, inhale deeply and say "Ah, yes!", then that essential oil is the one for you. Once you have found your oil, read its profile again carefully to check for any contraindications, and then look at the blends and methods I have given to help you to use it to its best effects.

Although this method of "following your nose" may seem simplistic, I have used it successfully countless times with my clients, throughout my years as an aromatherapist, to hone the choice of essential oils for a blend. If I follow a client's instinctive, positive reactions to the natural fragrances I put before them, I can be much more confident that I will see positive results from the treatment. On the whole, none of us is used to trusting our sense of smell, yet it is a powerful tool. Many of my clients have experienced profound inner healing because they have made instinctive choices about which essential oils I should use for them. As one woman says, "It's a sort of personal alchemy."

Over the following pages I will introduce you to the essential-oil groupings in more detail. This information provides a ready-reference to help you to find the selection of oils that are most relevant for you at any given time. It will also give you a sense of how the oils work to give specific effects, as well as some case studies of the successes that they have had in the past.

Muscle Treats

If you need to ease away general aches and pains, turn to the Muscle Treats group of oils (pp.100–121). They are strong-smelling and quickly boost the circulation under the skin, which warms the muscles, brings fresh blood to the tissues and helps to flush away toxins. They will also help if you suffer from rheumatism or osteoarthritis. The aromas of these oils are energizing and enlivening; they are full of fresh aromatic notes that lift the spirits.

Muscle Treats essential oils

The following oils are featured in the Muscle Treats section. See the individual entries for blend suggestions.

Silver Fir (p.100), Cypress (p.102), Lemongrass (p.104), Lavandin (p.106), Spike Lavender (p.108), Scots Pine (p.110), Rosemary (p.112), Spanish Sage (p.114), Vetiver (p.116), Plai (p.118), Ginger (p.120)

Energizing the muscles

Some years ago I had the privilege of massaging an American Olympic middle-distance runner. She asked me to use a blend that included Rosemary essential oil, because she said that it helped to warm her muscles before she ran and she knew that her body responded positively to its effects. Rosemary (pp.112–13) is a wonderful Muscle Treat oil – it energizes the muscles and prepares them for action. When my client used my blend, applying it before every race, she felt that her running was more fluid and powerful.

Skin Enhancers

The skin-enhancing oils in Part Two (see pp.122–147) provide a variety of properties that will clear, revitalize and rejuvenate the complexion, as well as help to heal many skin problems, such as eczema, dermatitis and itchy skin. The rejuvenating benefits of these oils come from the fact that they work in the various layers of the skin to encourage healthy cell renewal.

Skin Enhancers essential oils

The following oils appear in the Skin Enhancers section. See the individual profiles for suggested face blends, mousses and skin-healing formulae.

Yarrow (p.122), Roman Chamomile (p.124), Frankincense (p.126), Elemi (p.128), Orange Leaf (p.130), Bergamot (p.132), Lavender (p.134), German Chamomile (p.136), Tea Tree (p.138), Moroccan Chamomile (p.140), Geranium (p.142), Rose Geranium (p.144), Patchouli (p.146)

Help for damaged hands

One of my clients persuaded her husband to come to see me. He was a furniture restorer who used chemicals and varnishes at work. His hands were in a terrible state, with deep cracks in the skin and extreme dryness. I made a thick oil-based treatment using 5 drops each of German Chamomile (pp.136–7) and Myrrh (pp.150–51) in 20g/4 tsp carrier oil. I asked him to apply the salve every evening. After only two weeks, his lesions had healed and his skin no longer looked "papery" – it was a normal, healthy pink again.

Easy Breathers

Penetrating, fresh and medicinal-smelling, the essential oils in the Easy Breathers group (see pp.148–169) all clear problems in the respiratory system resulting from colds, flu, sinusitis and hay fever. The expectorant effects of these essential oils open the air passages to make breathing much easier.

Easy Breathers essential oils

Choose essential oils from this group to use in vaporizers, inhalations or baths, or in blends for chest massage. See the individual profiles for a range of effective combinations.

Himalayan Cedarwood (p.148), Myrrh (p.150), Lemon-scented Eucalyptus (p.152), Eucalyptus (p.154), Laurel Leaf (p.156), Cajeput (p.158), Niaouli (p.160), Myrtle (p.162), Black Spruce (p.164), Benzoin Resinoid (p.166), Thyme (p.168)

Treating a chesty cough

A friend's eight-year-old son was suffering from a chesty cough that kept him awake at night. I made him a simple blend of 2 drops each of Lemon-scented Eucalyptus (pp.152–3) and Myrtle (pp.162–3) in 20ml/4 tsp carrier oil. I advised my friend to rub the blend into her son's chest twice a day, and to vaporize Himalayan Cedarwood (pp.148–9) by his bed at night to help him to breathe. He recovered in a week.

Warming Stimulants

This group (see pp.170–79) of warming, spicy oils works wonders by easing away stiffness in the body and stimulating the circulation to keep us warm from the inside, especially in the winter. The oils are also fantastic for cold hands, feet or limbs at any time of year, bringing a sense of tingling warmth and energy. They also help to alleviate feelings of physical tiredness.

Warming Stimulants essential oils

The following oils are featured in the Warming Stimulants section. They work brilliantly in blends for body massage, especially when applied with vigorous strokes, and kneading. See the individual profiles for some great combinations.

Cinnamon Leaf (p.170), West Indian Bay (p.172), Cubeb Seed (p.174), Black Pepper (p.176), Clove Bud (p.178)

Warming cold feet

A client had icy-cold feet that never seemed to warm up. I advised her to soak them each evening in a warm footbath containing 2 drops Black Pepper (pp.176–7). I also made her a blend using 6 drops Black Pepper and 4 drops Cinnamon Leaf (pp.170–71) in 20ml/4 tsp carrier oil to use for a foot massage after the footbath. After three weeks of soaking and massaging her feet every night, my client found that her feet felt totally revived – and, crucially, they felt warm. She said that they felt better than they ever had before!

Immune Boosters

Great allies of our immune system, the wonderful essential oils in the Immune Boosters group (see pp.180–197) help the body to fight viral infections and ease the symptoms of conditions such as post-viral fatigue. You can also use them regularly throughout the colder months in aromatic baths or massage to help to prevent the onset of colds and flu.

Immune Boosters essential oils

Choose from this group of oils to make blends for massage, baths and inhalations that will strengthen your immune system. See the individual profiles for the most effective combinations.

Linaloe Wood (p.180), Lemon (p.182), Immortelle (p.184), Kanuka (p.186), Lemon Tea Tree (p.188), Manuka (p.190), Black Cumin Seed (p.192), Ravensara (p.194), Spanish Marjoram (p.196)

Fighting flu

I always treat myself with essential oils to speed my recovery from flu. As soon as the illness hits, I use 2 drops each of Manuka (pp.190–91) and Ravensara (pp.194–5) in my evening bath, and I make a blend combining 2 drops Black Cumin Seed (pp.192–3), 2 drops Manuka and 6 drops Lemon (pp.182–3) in a carrier oil, which I then massage into my chest and throat every night and morning. I find that these two methods used together help me to recover in just a week or so.

Hormone Harmonizers

Some oils are able to help to balance the female hormone cycle, easing symptoms such as fluid retention and mood swings. The Hormone Harmonizers (see pp.198–211) include plants that have mild oestrogen-enhancing effects, such as Fennel (see pp.200–201), which is good for period problems (including pre-menstrual syndrome/PMS) and the menopause. Try combining oils from this group with those from Uplifting Aromas (see pp.250–75) to make physically and emotionally supportive massage blends.

Hormone Harmonizers essential oils

The following essential oils are featured in the Hormone Harmonizers section.

Palmarosa (p.198), Fennel (p.200), Juniper Berry (p.202), Sweet Marjoram (p.204), Clary Sage (p.206), Australian Sandalwood (p.208), Agnus Castus (p.210)

Helping to overcome severe PMS

A client came to me with a combination of debilitating PMS symptoms, including headaches, low energy levels and mood swings. I made her a blend containing 4 drops Sweet Marjoram (pp.204–5), 2 drops Fennel (pp.200–201) and 4 drops Australian Sandalwood (pp.208–9) in 20ml/4 tsp carrier oil and suggested that she massage it into her abdomen every day during the last week of her cycle. After four months, her PMS symptoms had become much more manageable – she had more energy and felt generally more positive.

Nerve Relievers

The Nerve Relievers group of essential oils (see pp.212–225) helps to ease problems of the nervous system, such as tiredness, insomnia, anxiety and depression. We have all, at times, felt the build-up of mental and emotional stress that can lead to burnout and exhaustion. With their sedative and calming properties, the oils in this group help the body to cope better with stress and to experience quality relaxation. Some of these oils are known as "euphoric", meaning that they bring about positive moods.

Nerve Relievers essential oils

Choose from the following essential oils when your nervous system is in need of a boost. Look at the individual profiles for some soothing blends.

Citronella (p.212), May Chang (p.214), Nutmeg (p.216), Sweet Basil (p.218), Tulsi or Indian Holy Basil (p.220), Damiana (p.222), Valerian (p.224)

De-stressing a workaholic
One of my clients was suffering from insomnia. After initial consultations, it was clear that he was unable to switch off from work in the evenings – he even kept his laptop going until the moment he switched off the light to go to sleep. I advised him to have an evening aromatherapy bath with 4 drops May Chang (pp.214–15) and 2 drops Valerian (pp.224–5), and also to vaporize these oils beside his bed. A combination of using these aromatherapy methods and slightly changing his evening routine dramatically helped to improve his sleep.

Digestive Soothers

Pungent and uplifting, the Digestive Soothers (see pp.226–249) include many oils derived from fruits and herbs, such as citrus oils and types of mint. These oils' aromas often cause the stomach to rumble – a sign that they are stimulating the digestive system. Digestive Soothers can help to ease problems such as indigestion, constipation, bloating and irritable bowel syndrome (IBS).

Digestive Soothers essential oils

The following oils all feature in the Digestive Soothers section. Try applying them using abdomen massage – in a circular, clockwise movement.

Angelica Root (p.226), Grapefruit (p.228), Tangerine (p.230), Sweet Orange (p.232), Coriander Seed (p.234), Turmeric (p.236), Carrot Seed (p.238), Cardamom (p.240), Lovage Root (p.242), Peppermint (p.244), Bergamot Mint (p.246), Spearmint (p.248)

Massaging away stress and IBS

A client with a stressful job came to me complaining of IBS, characterized by tension in her abdomen and bouts of constipation. I gave her weekly massage sessions over eight weeks, using 2 drops Turmeric (pp.236–7), 4 drops Sweet Orange (pp.232–3) and 4 drops Cardamom (pp.240–41) in a carrier. She also used this blend to massage her own abdomen every evening. Her stress levels fell, her constipation eased away and her mood improved dramatically.

Uplifting Aromas

The oils in the Uplifting Aromas group (see pp.250–275) are the most glorious of all: the best tools to soothe away emotional anxiety. As well as having long-lasting scents that combine easily for many different effects, they enhance many of my suggested blends throughout Part Two, adding an extra level of relaxation and uplifting energy. Many of these oils are precious gifts given to us by flowers; they represent Nature at its most exquisite and subtle.

Uplifting Aromas essential oils

The following essential oils fall into the Uplifting Aromas section.

Ylang Ylang (p.250), Cistus (p.252), Lime (p.254), Neroli (p.256), Mandarin (p.258), Jasmine Absolute (p.260), Melissa (p.262), Spikenard (p.264), Rose Absolute (p.266), Rose Otto (p.268), Linden Blossom Absolute (p.270), Vanilla Absolute (p.272), Violet Leaf Absolute (p.274)

Healing the heart

I met a woman who was feeling very low after her relationship with her partner had broken down. I massaged her on a weekly basis for two months with a blend of 4 drops Rose Otto (pp.268–9), 4 drops Mandarin (pp.258–9) and 2 drops Spikenard (pp.264–5). Every time I massaged her she said that she felt "enfolded" by the aroma: as soon as she smelled it, the Rose Otto oil made her feel safe and at peace. She began to relax very deeply, which in turn helped her painful inner feelings to begin to heal.

Making the most of the guide

The next part of this book is a guide to 100 oils. The first 12 of these are carrier oils, some basic carriers (see pp.76–83) and others, called Skin Foods, with specific skin-nourishing effects (see pp.84–99). You should use these oils as the bases for any blend that you make, unless I instruct otherwise in the blend boxes. Mostly, it is up to you which carrier you choose – read up on their properties and choose one that suits your skin type or particular needs.

The remaining 88 oils are essential oils. For each oil entry I give some background information about the oil, how it is extracted and what it smells like. Then, I give important safety information and details on ways in which you can use the essential oils to therapeutic effect for mind, body and spirit.

It is crucial that you read all the safety information for any oil that you select to ensure that it is suitable for your skin type and that it is not contraindicated in any other way. The same goes for any other oils in a blend: all the given blends are made up of oils that feature in the book, so you should look up the safety information for each one before making and applying the blend. It is worth reiterating here that, other than Lavender and Tea Tree, you should *never* use essential oils undiluted on your skin, and that for all essential oils you must use them only according to the numbers of drops stated in each blend (half that amount if you have sensitive skin, or if you are pregnant and none of the oils in the blend is contraindicated).

While it is important to keep safety in mind when using essential oils, it's important also to remember that aromatherapy should be fun. Enjoy exploring this fragrant world – experiment with the oils and their scents, find the ones you love best and then use them whenever you can.

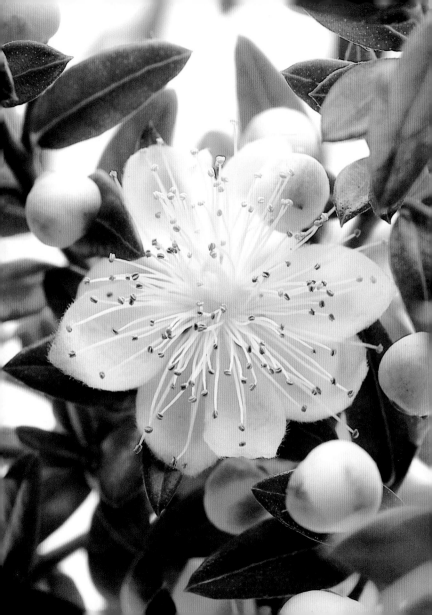

Part Two:
A Guide to Oils

In this part of the book we bring you a directory of no less than 100 oils. The first 12 of these are carrier oils – these include four basic carriers, which you'll need as bases to make aromatherapy blends, and eight special "skin-food" carrier oils, which can enrich a massage base when your skin needs particular care. To make it easy for you to source the oils that are right for you, we have grouped all subsequent 88 essential oils into special "treatment" categories. So, if you need to speed your recovery from a virus, turn to the Immune Boosters; if you have a strain or sprain, or you ache from pent-up stress, turn to the Muscle Treats; and so on. Each oil entry presents all the information you need to select and use that oil, including safety information, notes on its aroma and ideas on how to use it in blends for specific effects on your mind, body and spirit.

Sunflower *(Helianthus annuus)*

The sunflower's botanical name derives from the Greek word *helios*, meaning "sun". The seeds of the giant flower (which is the largest member of the daisy family) contain about 40-per-cent oil. This oil is light-textured, yet nourishing to the skin. Avoid processed, supermarket-grade oil and instead choose unrefined organic oil, as it contains skin-enhancing ingredients, such as potassium, vitamins B and E, and omega-6 fatty acids.

Plant features: Large flower with yellow petals

Part of plant used: Seeds

Oil produced in: Australia, Argentina, Hungary

Extraction method: Pressing

Safety first
Sunflower oil is safe for all skin types.

Facial nourishment
- Sunflower oil softens the face without leaving a residue (see first blend, opposite).
- This carrier protects and restores combination skins. Apply it to your face mixed with Geranium, Roman Chamomile and Linaloe Wood (second blend, opposite).

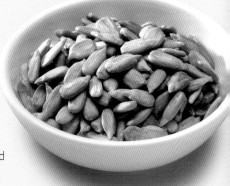

76

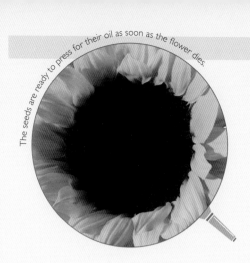

The seeds are ready to press for their oil as soon as the flower dies.

Keywords

Light

Soothing

• Sunflower oil is ideal for complexions that do not require intensive nourishment.

Body treatment
• This is a superb all-round massage oil.
• The vitamin-F content of sunflower oil helps to heal blemishes and improve scar tissue.

Special tip
To repair damaged hair that has split ends, massage 40ml/8 tsp sunflower oil into dry hair, from the roots to the tips. Leave the oil in for 20 minutes, then, without wetting your hair, massage in an unfragranced shampoo, and rinse. Your hair will feel silky smooth.

Special blends

Add these essential oils to 20ml/4 tsp Sunflower carrier oil:

To soften and nourish tired-looking, dry skin:
4 drops Australian Sandalwood, 2 drops Patchouli, 4 drops Sweet Orange

To soothe combination skin:
4 drops Geranium, 2 drops Roman Chamomile, 4 drops Linaloe Wood

Apricot Kernel (*Prunus armeniaca*)

This carrier comes from the kernels of the apricot fruit. Originally native to Armenia (which gives us the botanical name), Apricot Kernel carrier oil is now produced all over the southern Mediterranean, in particular in Turkey and Spain. The fruit is a valuable source of beta-carotene, which the body converts to vitamin A, an important immune-booster and skin-nourisher. The carrier oil is produced by crushing the kernels, and the yield is very rich in oleic acid, a nourishing fatty-acid compound also found in olive oil. This compound is the main reason why Apricot Kernel oil is so good at smoothing the skin and improving its texture.

Safety first
Apricot Kernel carrier is safe for all skin types.

Facial nourishment
• Apricot Kernel oil rehydrates dry skin, especially when it is inflamed by the sun or wind. Try massaging it into your face mixed with Neroli, Frankincense and Roman Chamomile (see first blend, right).

Plant features: Small tree with orange fruit

Part of plant used: Kernels of fruit

Oil produced in: Turkey, Spain

Extraction method: Pressing

Special blends

Add these essential oils to 20ml/4 tsp Apricot Kernel oil:

To moisturize dry skin on the face:
4 drops Neroli, 2 drops Frankincense, 4 drops Roman Chamomile

To nourish dry skin in body massage:
6 drops Australian Sandalwood, 2 drops Palmarosa, 2 drops Mandarin

- This carrier oil replenishes and rejuvenates mature skin.

Keywords

Calming

Rejuvenating

Body treatment

- Apricot Kernel oil is excellent to massage into dry, poorly nourished skin anywhere on the body. Try it mixed with Australian Sandalwood, Palmarosa and Mandarin (see second blend, left).
- This carrier helps to soothe minor skin irritations or mild eczema.
- This oil helps to repair areas of extra-dry skin (see below).

Special tip

If you have dry elbows, take two small bowls and place 20ml/4 tsp Apricot Kernel oil in each one. After a bath or shower, when your skin is still moist, place your elbows in the bowls and soak for at least 5 minutes. Pat off any excess oil to reveal wonderfully soft skin.

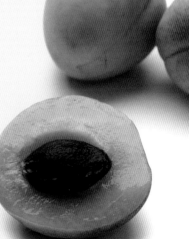

79

Sweet Almond (*Prunus dulcis* syn. *Prunus amygdalus*)

Pressed from the edible nuts of the sweet almond tree, Sweet Almond oil is rich in both minerals and oleic acid, a skin-nourisher and hydrator. In Mediterranean countries, where the tree is native, Sweet Almond oil is used to treat dryness, chapped hands and sun-damaged skin. This carrier has a slippery feel, so you will need to massage it thoroughly into your skin. Once you have, the surface of your skin will improve dramatically, feeling smooth and silky.

Plant features: Small tree with pink flowers

Part of plant used: Nuts

Oil produced in: Spain, Turkey

Extraction method: Pressing

Safety first
Do not use Sweet Almond oil if you suffer from a nut allergy.

Facial nourishment
- Sweet Almond oil softens undernourished or dry skin, encouraging cell renewal. Try it with Rose Otto, Neroli and Frankincense (see first blend, opposite).
- This oil rejuvenates the skin and reduces fine lines.

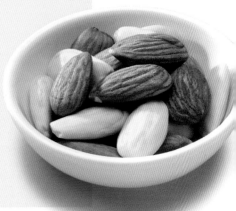

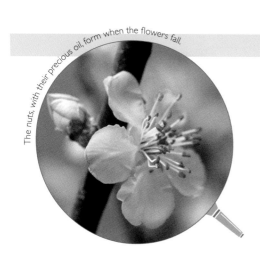

The nuts, with their precious oil, form when the flowers fall.

Keywords

Nourishing

Softening

Body treatment

- Sweet Almond oil lubricates the skin well, allowing for smooth massage movements.
- This oil moisturizes dry or baby skin.
- If you have cracked skin on your heels or elbows, this oil will aid healing. Rub it in mixed with Myrrh, German Chamomile and Patchouli (see second blend, right).

Special tip

For dry hands or damaged nails, stand the base of a small glass dish of 100ml/3¹/₂ fl oz Sweet Almond oil in a bowl of hot water to warm the oil (this improves absorption). Then soak your hands or nails in the warmed oil for 10 minutes.

Special blends

Add these essential oils to 20ml/4 tsp Sweet Almond oil:

To rehydrate dry skin:
2 drops Rose Otto, 4 drops Neroli, 4 drops Frankincense

To rejuvenate scaly skin on the heels and elbows:
4 drops Myrrh, 4 drops German Chamomile, 2 drops Patchouli

81

Grapeseed *(Vitis vinifera)*

Grapeseed oil is pressed from the pips of grapes, as a by-product of wine-making. The oil is pale green and extremely high in polyunsaturated fatty acids, making it light-textured and easy for the skin to absorb; it also has useful skin-softening properties. This oil has to be slightly refined before we can use it in cooking or massage as the crude oil has an unpleasant odour. However, this processing does not affect the oil's beneficial properties. Grapeseed comes into its own when massaged into complexions that are well-lubricated, such as olive or darker skins, which have higher levels of their own natural oils. These skin-types tend not to absorb richer carriers, resulting in very slippery skin. Massaging with a very light carrier such as Grapeseed leaves no residue and creates a lovely smooth finish.

Safety first

Grapeseed oil is completely safe for all skin types. In aromatherapy practice, Grapeseed is often used as a safe carrier for people who suffer from nut allergies.

Plant features:
Grape-producing vine

Part of plant used:
Pips of fruit

Oil produced in:
France, Spain

Extraction method:
Pressing

Special blends

Add these essential oils to 20ml/4 tsp Grapeseed oil:

To tone normal and oily skins:
2 drops Cypress,
6 drops Grapefruit,
2 drops Fennel

To smooth normal skin:
4 drops Lavender,
4 drops Lemon,
2 drops Vetiver

Facial nourishment

Grapeseed oil softens normal, oily and combination skins. Try massaging it into your face mixed with Cypress, Grapefruit and Fennel (see first blend, left).

Keywords

Silky

Softening

Body treatment

- This carrier helps to maintain the silkiness of normal skin and enables the smooth flow of massage movements over all skin-types. Try it in a body massage mixed with Lavender, Lemon and Vetiver (see second blend, left).
- Grapeseed oil makes a fantastic, light body moisturizer for combination skins.

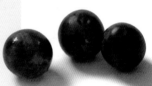

Special tip

To smooth away hard skin on your feet, use a Grapeseed and sea-salt foot scrub. Place 90ml/3 fl oz Grapeseed oil in a small bowl and add 25g/1 tbsp coarse sea salt. After a bath or shower, rub the foot scrub all over both feet, then wipe away any excess.

83

Kukui Nut (*Aleurites moluccana*)

The Kukui tree has many restorative powers – for example, the sap can be used to heal chapped skin, and the beautiful, heart-shaped nuts (a symbol of love in Hawaii) can be roasted, then pounded into a paste and applied to wounds, rheumatic joints and aching backs. Hawaiian mothers apply the oil to newborn babies – it protects their skin from dryness and prevents dehydration. You can use Kukui Nut as a base for essential oil blends, or on its own to treat specific skin problems, such as eczema or psoriasis. As it is more expensive than other carriers, for an enriched base, use 1 part Kukui to 3 parts basic carrier (see pp.76–83).

Safety first

There are no reported safety issues with Kukui Nut oil, but avoid it if you have a nut allergy.

Facial nourishment

Kukui restructures mature skin, improving texture. Try it mixed with a basic carrier oil and Neroli, Australian Sandalwood and Patchouli essential oils (see first blend, right).

Plant features:
Nut tree

Part of plant used:
Nuts

Oil produced in:
Hawaii, West Pacific

Extraction method:
Pressing

Special blends

Add these essential oils to 15ml/3 tsp basic carrier oil (see pp.76–83) plus 5ml/1 tsp Kukui Nut oil:

To nourish mature skin:
2 drops Neroli, 4 drops Australian Sandalwood, 4 drops Patchouli

To soothe eczema or psoriasis:
4 drops Yarrow, 4 drops Palmarosa, 2 drops Frankincense

Body treatment

- Kukui Nut heals eczema, especially areas that are deeply cracked, and restructures skin that has been damaged by psoriasis. Try it mixed with a basic carrier and Yarrow, Palmarosa and Frankincense (see second blend, left) and apply it to the affected areas.
- This oil regenerates extremely dry skin. Massage it in well on a daily basis where your skin needs it most.

Special tip

Kukui Nut is superb on its own for baby massage, particularly if your baby suffers from eczema or very dry skin. Unlike commercial baby oil, which forms a barrier over the skin, Kukui works within the skin's layers to create a stronger and more supple skin texture. Warm 5ml/1 tsp oil in your hands and rub it gently into your baby's skin. (If you are worried about nut allergies, do a patch test first; see p.25.)

Keywords

Regenerating

Skin-healing

85

Aloe Vera *(Aloe vera)*

Known for its medicinal properties for more than a thousand years, the aloe vera plant was originally native to parts of East and South Africa, but was introduced to the West Indies in the 17th century and has flourished there ever since. Aloe is a succulent plant with no stem, just fleshy leaves containing special sacs filled with a healing juice. Fresh from the plant, this juice can be applied to burns, cuts, wounds and sunburn with rapid anti-inflammatory and skin-healing results. Commercial production extracts the juice and thickens it into a gel. Always buy products that are at least 90-per-cent pure aloe vera for the best healing effects.

Safety first

Aloe Vera gel is safe for all skin types.

Facial nourishment

- Aloe Vera calms angry red skin.
- The gel cools skin reactions resulting from sensitivity or allergy.
- Aloe Vera heals skin that has been affected by eczema, psoriasis or shingles (caused by

Plant features: Succulent plant, thick leaves	
Part of plant used: Gel from leaves	
Oil produced in: West Indies, USA, Canary Islands	
Extraction method: Cutting open the leaves	

Special blends

Add these essential oils to 20g/4 tsp Aloe Vera gel:

To heal eczema or to soothe inflamed skin:
4 drops Yarrow, 4 drops Neroli, 2 drops Patchouli

To soothe sunburn:
4 drops Lavender, 2 drops Rose Otto, 4 drops Roman Chamomile

the Herpes zoster virus). Mix it with Yarrow,
Neroli and Patchouli (see first blend, left) and
apply it to the affected areas.

Keywords

Cooling

Soothing

Body treatment

• Apply the gel directly to ease burns or
sunburn, and infected cuts or wounds. You
could also mix it with Lavender, Rose Otto
and Roman Chamomile (see second blend,
left) to make a particularly cooling, soothing
ointment for sore patches of sunburn.

• Use Aloe Vera in a Skin Mousse (see
pp.42–3) to heal dehydrated skin, or rashes.

Special tip

Use this gel with hydrating honey to make a
calming face mask for reddened, dry skin
that has been exposed to the sun or
wind. Mix 10g/2 tsp Aloe Vera gel
with 5ml/1 tsp good-quality honey.
Apply the mixture to your face
and leave it for 10 minutes.
Then wash it off with
warm water and pat dry.

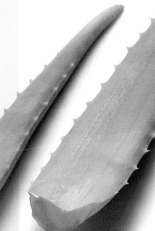

87

Borage Seed (*Borago officinalis*)

Valued as a remedy for depression by the 16th-century English herbalist John Gerard, borage grows wild in woodland and on grassy banks in the European countryside. Its silky stems and leaves are covered in tiny hairs, and in summer it displays beautiful star-shaped, blue flowers, which is why Borage Seed oil is sometimes called Starflower oil. The seeds of these flowers yield a vegetable oil that is rich in skin-nourishing fatty acids and is often sold in capsules as a nutritional supplement. To provide extra nourishment to dry skin, make a wonderfully enriched massage base by piercing one large capsule and squeezing the oil into 20ml/4 tsp basic carrier.

Plant features: Shrub with blue star-shaped flowers

Part of plant used:
Seeds

Oil produced in:
UK, US

Extraction method:
Pressing

Safety first
Borage Seed (or Starflower) oil is safe for all skin types.

Facial nourishment
• Borage Seed oil replenishes and restores dry, wrinkled or ageing skin. Mix it with Rose

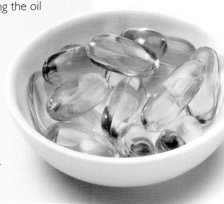

Otto, Jasmine Absolute and Frankincense
(see first blend, right) and apply the blend
when you need it most.
- This carrier oil encourages the renewal of
skin cells for a more supple complexion.
- Borage Seed oil calms and soothes sensitive
skin. Apply it at least twice a day.

Body treatment
- To restore and rehydrate extremely dry
skin, apply Borage Seed oil in a blend with
Australian Sandalwood, Geranium and
Palmarosa (see second blend, right).
- This oil is wonderful for repairing areas of
damaged skin, such as on the heels or elbows.

Special tip
Borage Seed is an excellent nighttime nourisher
for the face. Pierce one large capsule (1000iu)
of the oil and apply it to your face just before
you go to bed, using tiny, circular movements
with your fingers, and patting it in gently with
the fingertips around the edges of your eyes
where your skin is particularly delicate.

Keywords

Replenishing

Renewing

Special blends

Add these essential oils
to 20ml/4 tsp basic
carrier oil (see pp.76–
83) and the contents of
1 pierced large (1000iu)
Borage Seed oil capsule.

**To rejuvenate
mature skin:**
4 drops Rose Otto, 2
drops Jasmine Absolute,
4 drops Frankincense

To rehydrate dry skin:
6 drops Australian
Sandalwood, 2 drops
Geranium, 2 drops
Palmarosa

89

Camellia *(Camellia sasanqua)*

In Japan, this species of Camellia (a type of tea bush) is celebrated as one of the first flowers to bloom in spring. The plant's fruit contains an extremely oily seed – the source of the carrier oil. In Japan, China and other parts of the Far East, Camellia oil has been used for centuries not only as a traditional hair conditioner, combed through to create long, silky tresses, but also as a treatment to nourish the complexion and strengthen brittle nails. Camellia is a wonderful, fine-textured carrier oil, which the skin absorbs immediately to leave a perfectly smooth finish. It is a rare and expensive oil, so if you can't use it on its own, add 1 part Camellia to 3 parts basic carrier oil (see pp.76–83) for an enriched massage base.

Safety first
Camellia oil is safe for all skin types.

Facial nourishment
- Camellia refines mature skin. Massage it into your face with Myrrh, Himalayan Cedarwood and Rose Absolute (see first blend, right).

Plant features: Small bush with small white flowers

Part of plant used: Kernels of seeds

Oil produced in: Japan, UK

Extraction method: Pressing

Special blends

Add these essential oils to 20ml/4 tsp Camellia oil; or to 15ml/3 tsp basic carrier oil (see pp.76–83) plus 5ml/1 tsp Camellia:

To smooth out mature skin:
2 drops Myrrh, 4 drops Himalayan Cedarwood, 4 drops Rose Absolute

To enhance normal skin:
4 drops Rose Geranium, 2 drops Mandarin, 4 drops Linaloe Wood

90

- Camellia strengthens normal and oily skins, soaking in entirely to leave no residue.
- This carrier oil rejuvenates tired or dry-looking skin. It's a perfect morning skin tonic as it's not greasy, meaning that you can apply make-up on top.

Body treatment

- Camellia helps to maintain balance in normal or naturally supple skins. Massage it in mixed with Rose Geranium, Mandarin, and Linaloe Wood (see second blend, left).
- This oil encourages cell renewal and, rubbed into the body, gives the skin an even texture.

Special tip

If you have long hair, try the following simple, natural treatment. After drying your hair, comb a small amount of Camellia oil through it, especially into the ends. You will find that this carrier is not greasy at all; it is simply absorbed into the hair shafts, creating a soft sheen.

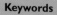

Keywords

Smoothing

Enhancing

91

Macadamia Nut *(Macadamia integrifolia)*

Macadamia nut trees are native to Australia, thriving in Queensland's humid rainforests. The whitish kernels inside the nuts contain up to 80-per-cent oil, a high yield that has led to commercial cultivation in other countries such as Hawaii, as well as parts of southern Europe. Macadamia Nut oil is rich in palmitoleic acid, which is similar to the skin's natural oil, sebum. Applying Macadamia Nut oil to baby skin or older, drier skin, where sebum production is lower, has dramatic moisturizing effects.

Plant features: Rainforest tree with white flowers

Part of plant used: Nuts

Oil produced in: Australia, Hawaii

Extraction method: Pressing

Safety first

Macadamia Nut oil is safe for all skin types, but avoid it if you suffer from a nut allergy.

Facial nourishment

- Macadamia Nut oil deeply moisturizes older, drier complexions. Massage it in with Neroli, Immortelle and Australian Sandalwood (see first blend, opposite).

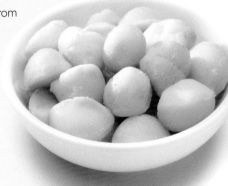

• This oil helps to repair skin damage resulting from exposure to the sun or wind.

Body treatment
• Macadamia Nut oil conditions very dry skin and nourishes slack-looking skin. Apply it using firm strokes to penetrate the skin well.
• This carrier repairs hardened or damaged skin on, for example, the knees, elbows, hands and feet (see below). Apply it regularly.

Special tip
Macadamia oil is wonderful for foot massage on extremely dry or hard skin. Try it mixed with Elemi, Myrrh and Spearmint (see second blend, right). Every night spend five minutes on each foot, rubbing in the blend after a bath or shower. Work from heel to toe along the sole of each foot, concentrating on any hard areas, usually around the heel and ball of the foot. Then rub in the blend from your ankle to your toes on the tops of your feet, and then all round your ankles. After only a few applications, cracks will heal and your skin will feel softer.

Keywords

Moisturizing

Softening

Special blends

Add these essential oils to 20ml/4 tsp Macadamia Nut oil:

To rejuvenate dry or wrinkled skin:
2 drops Neroli, 2 drops Immortelle, 6 drops Australian Sandalwood

To heal dry skin, paricularly on the feet:
2 drops Elemi,
4 drops Myrrh,
4 drops Spearmint

93

Evening Primrose (Oenothera biennis)

Despite its name, evening primrose is not a primrose at all, but a tall flower with a bright yellow bloom that opens in the evening to attract pollinators. The plant is native to Mexico and the US, but in the 17th century the English naturalist John Tradescant brought the plant back from North America to the UK, where it gradually naturalized itself. Evening Primrose oil is pressed from the plant's seeds. Rich in fatty acids, this oil is often taken as a nutritional supplement. However, you can also apply it to the skin as a nourishing treatment, particularly on the face. As it is expensive, add the contents of 1 large capsule to 20ml/4 tsp basic carrier oil for body massage.

Plant features: Tall plant with a bright yellow flower

Part of plant used: Seeds

Oil produced in: UK, US

Extraction method: Pressing

Safety first
This oil is safe for all skin types.

Facial nourishment
• Massage Evening Primrose oil into the face to encourage cell renewal in mature or wrinkled skin.

94

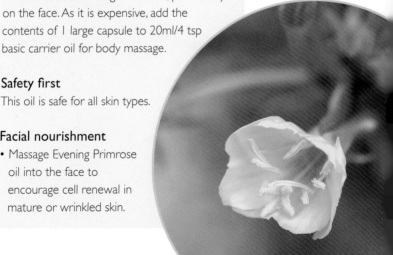

- Apply this oil to heal facial blemishes and improve skin texture.
- Evening Primrose oil will revitalize and strengthen skin cells on the face.

Body treatment

- This oil, like most "skin foods", restores suppleness to very dry skin. Massage it into dry patches daily mixed with Linaloe Wood, Palmarosa and Neroli (see first blend, right).
- Evening Primrose will help to soothe and heal the sore skin associated with eczema. Apply it to affected areas mixed with Yarrow, Roman Chamomile and Lavender (see second blend, right).

Special tip

For a special anti-wrinkle treatment, pierce a large Evening Primrose capsule (1000iu) and squeeze the oil into your palms. Apply it to your face, concentrating on areas that are particularly prone to lines, such as the forehead, the corners of your mouth and the outer edges of your eyes.

Keywords

Replenishing

Restoring

Special blends

Add these essential oils to 20ml/4 tsp basic carrier oil (see pp.76–83) and the contents of 1 large (1000iu) capsule of Evening Primrose oil.

To hydrate very dry skin:
4 drops Linaloe Wood,
4 drops Palmarosa,
2 drops Neroli

To soothe eczema:
4 drops Yarrow, 2 drops Roman Chamomile,
4 drops Lavender

95

Avocado (*Persea americana*)

In Mexico and Arizona, the oil from the flesh of the avocado pear has been used as a beauty treatment for hundreds of years. It is rich green as it still contains chlorophyll (the pigment that gives plants their hue). Avocados contain the skin-nourishing vitamins A and D, as well as linoleic acid, which strengthens cell walls, making the skin stronger. On its own, this oil is viscous and absorbs slowly into the skin, so it is difficult to apply in massage. However, if you combine Avocado with lighter oils (such as a basic carrier), using 1 part Avocado to 3 parts carrier, it provides a wonderful, rich emollient treatment for dry skin. It has been shown to slow down the signs of skin-ageing and even acts as a mild natural sunscreen.

Safety first
There are no safety issues with Avocado oil, so it is safe for all skin types.

Facial nourishment
- If you suffer from very dry skin on your face, apply Avocado oil mixed with Melissa, Rose

Plant features: Shrub with green fruit

Part of plant used: Flesh of fruit

Oil produced in: US, Mexico

Extraction method: Pressing

Special blends

Add these essential oils to 15ml/3 tsp basic carrier oil (see pp.76–83), plus 5ml/1 tsp Avocado oil:

To moisturize very dry skin:
2 drops Melissa, 4 drops Rose Geranium, 4 drops Tangerine

To soothe sunburn:
6 drops Lavender, 2 drops German Chamomile, 2 drops Yarrow

Geranium and Tangerine (see first blend, left), every morning and night.

- Avocado carrier oil nourishes complexions that have been depleted by the sun, heat or wind. Apply it as necessary mixed with Lavender, German Chamomile and Yarrow (see second blend, left).
- Applied nightly, this oil can slow down the degeneration of the skin and so help to reduce visible signs of ageing.

Keywords

Enriching

Deeply moisturizing

Body treatment
- Avocado provides intense moisturization for dry skin. Rub it into affected areas.
- Applied specifically, this oil repairs damaged skin, such as on the elbows, knees or heels.

Special tip
For split or damaged nails, soak the fingertips in 20ml/4 tsp pure Avocado oil for 10 minutes each night; wipe off any excess and then rub the nails really well to encourage absorption.

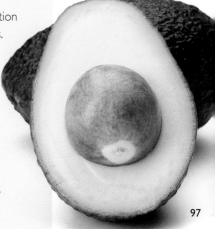

Jojoba *(Simmondsia chinensis)*

Beautiful, golden-yellow Jojoba oil (pronounced "ho-ho-ba") comes from the beans of a tough shrub native to the deserts of Mexico and Arizona. This carrier oil has been used by Native Americans for centuries to protect their skins from dehydration. It is actually a liquid wax that solidifies at cool temperatures, and is similar in composition to sebum, the skin's natural oil, so our skin is able to absorb it easily.

Plant features: Tough desert shrub

Part of plant used: Beans

Oil produced in: USA, Mexico

Extraction method: Pressing

Safety first

Jojoba oil is safe for all skin types.

Facial nourishment

- Jojoba strengthens sensitive skin. For a delicate facial treatment, apply it mixed with small amounts of Yarrow and Rose Otto in a low concentration (see first blend, opposite).
- Jojoba balances oily skin and clears acne and even long-term scars. Apply it to the affected areas mixed

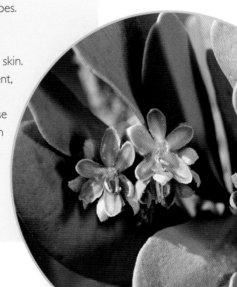

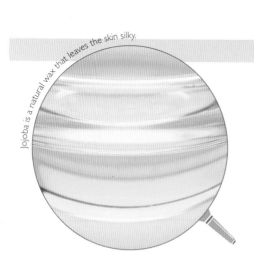

Jojoba is a natural wax that leaves the skin silky.

with Lemon, Frankincense and Ylang Ylang
(see second blend, right).

Body treatment

- Applied regularly, Jojoba softens and
  moisturizes dry, dehydrated or sensitive skin.
- This oil also helps to soothe and heal skin
  damaged by eczema or psoriasis, whether
  used on its own or as a blend.

Special tip

Jojoba is a great cleanser: its waxiness dissolves
away dirt and excess oils. Pour 2.5ml/¹/₂ tsp
onto an absorbent cotton wool pad and wipe
it over your face, morning and night.

Special blends

Add these essential oils
to 20ml/4 tsp Jojoba oil:

To soothe sensitive skin:
2 drops Yarrow, 2 drops
Rose Otto (note low
concentration)

**To tone oily skin,
reduce surface grease
and heal scars:**
4 drops Lemon, 4 drops
Frankincense, 2 drops
Ylang Ylang

99

Silver Fir (*Abies alba*)

A small, delicate tree with silvery-white bark and feathery foliage, the silver fir is native to the northern US and Canada, as well as many northern European countries, including Russia and Germany, where most Silver Fir essential oil is produced. The tree's bark secretes a pungent resin – Native Americans burned it both as incense in spiritual ceremonies and as a purifying antiseptic to fight infection. European herbal tradition still values the resin to help respiratory complaints, as well as muscular aches and pains. Silver Fir essential oil comes from the twigs and foliage and has a rich, sweet and slightly balsamic aroma, with pine notes.

Plant features:
Small evergreen fir tree

Part of plant used:
Leaves and twigs

Oil produced in: Russia, Germany, US, Canada

Extraction method:
Steam distillation

Safety first
• Silver Fir is non-toxic and non-irritant.
• Avoid Silver Fir if you are asthmatic, as its aroma may aggravate your sensitive airways.

Supporting the spirit
• This essential oil calms and deepens the breath, encouraging a sense of inner restoration and a feeling of space.

Special blends

Add these essential oils to 20ml/4 tsp carrier oil:

To ease stiffness:
4 drops Silver fir, 2 drops Ginger, 4 drops Spike Lavender

To relieve a tired body:
2 drops Silver Fir, 2 drops Vetiver, 6 drops Sweet Marjoram

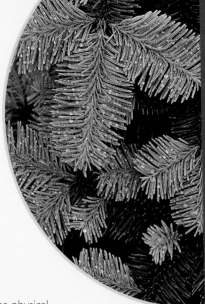

- This oil's aroma gives a sense of deep inner strength, building the courage to take action.

Easing the mind
- To relieve high levels of mental anxiety, try 3 drops Silver Fir and 3 drops Lavender in a bath.
- To clear the mind and improve concentration, vaporize 3 drops Silver Fir and 3 drops Eucalyptus.

Healing the body
- To loosen stiff muscles and release physical tension, blend Silver Fir with Ginger and Spike Lavender in a carrier oil (see first blend, left) and massage it into the sore areas.
- To ease physical tiredness, restore aching limbs and generally soothe your body, rub in a blend of Silver Fir, Vetiver and Sweet Marjoram in a carrier (see second blend, left).
- To ease chest congestion and catarrh, try an inhalation with 3 drops Silver Fir and 2 drops Himalayan Cedarwood.

Keywords
Warming
Soothing
Grounding

Cypress *(Cupressus sempervirens)*

Cypress trees belong to one of the oldest plant families on Earth – the *Cupressaceae*, which is some 17 million years old. The trees can live for many hundreds of years, which has given them the name *sempervirens*, meaning "ever-alive". In the folklore of many countries, cypress trees are seen as a gateway to the "otherworld" or the afterlife, which is why they are often found in churchyards. In Tibet, twigs and branches of this evergreen tree are burned as sacred incense. The essential oil is produced from the leaves and twigs, and has a deep, earthy and smoky aroma, with sharper fresh notes as it evaporates.

Plant features:
Tall, conical evergreen tree

Part of plant used:
Leaves and twigs

Oil produced in:
France, Spain

Extraction method:
Steam distillation

Safety first
Cypress essential oil is non-toxic, non-irritating and non-sensitizing, so is safe for all skin types.

Supporting the spirit
• Cypress acts like a spiritual plumb line, bridging the

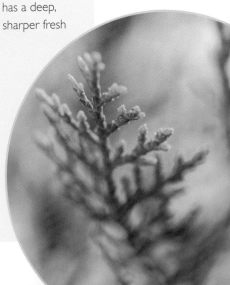

subtle and physical worlds and bringing the mind into balance with the spirit.

• This oil helps to develop inner wisdom.

Easing the mind

• To help to cope with life's transitions, such as leaving home or starting a new job, vaporize 2 drops Cypress and 4 drops Lemon.
• To calm overstretched emotions, take a bath with 2 drops Cypress and 4 drops Lavender.

Healing the body

• To ease spasms in overworked and tired muscles, mix Cypress, Ginger and Sweet Marjoram in a carrier oil (see first blend, right) and apply it to the sore areas.
• To remove toxins from muscles and reduce cellulite, blend Cypress with Grapefruit and Juniper Berry in a carrier oil (see second blend, right) and rub it into the affected parts.
• To cleanse oily skins, and to heal acne, add 4 drops Cypress, 2 drops Manuka and 4 drops Orange Leaf to 20g/4 tsp Skin Mousse (see pp.42–3) and apply it to your face.

Keywords

Strengthening

Earthy

Centring

Special blends

Add these essential oils to 20ml/4 tsp carrier oil:

To release muscle spasm:
4 drops Cypress, 2 drops Ginger, 4 drops Sweet Marjoram

To help to improve the appearance of cellulite:
4 drops Cypress, 4 drops Grapefruit, 2 drops Juniper Berry

103

Lemongrass *(Cymbopogon citratus)*

Fresh and sharp with a lemony fizz, the aroma of Lemongrass oil is instantly energizing. The oil comes from a fast-growing, scented Indian grass that reaches heights of up to 1.5m/3ft. In traditional Ayurvedic medicine, the grass is used to help to lower fevers and calm the nervous system. Because the plant and its essential oil have a strong, lemony scent, they are also both used to keep stinging insects at bay. Traditional Chinese Medicine recommends Lemongrass oil to ease stomach pains, and also to relieve headaches, colds and rheumatism.

Plant features:
Aromatic tropical grass

Part of plant used:
Young shoots

Oil produced in:
India, Guatemala

Extraction method:
Steam distillation

Safety first
- Lemongrass is non-toxic.
- Avoid using Lemongrass in baths or massage if you have sensitive or allergy-prone skin.
- This oil is a moderate irritant. Even if you have normal skin, use a maximum of 2 drops Lemongrass in the bath as it can sting.

Supporting the spirit

- Lemongrass oil cuts through any emotional fog and will help you to see things clearly.
- Like a ray of sunshine, this oil relieves depression and encourages positivity.

Easing the mind

- To clear mental clutter and improve your powers of concentration, place 1 drop Lemongrass on a tissue and inhale.
- To chase away bad dreams or insomnia, vaporize 2 drops Lemongrass with 2 drops Lavender in an electric vaporizer as you sleep.

Healing the body

- To ease muscular aches, muscle spasm or physical tension, mix Lemongrass with Ginger and Lavandin in a carrier oil (see first blend, right) and rub it into the affected areas.
- To soothe indigestion or help to relieve constipation, mix Lemongrass with Coriander Seed and Mandarin in a carrier oil (see second blend, right) and apply it twice a day, using clockwise abdominal massage.

Keywords

Zesty

Fresh

Invigorating

Special blends

Add these essential oils to 20ml/4 tsp carrier oil:

To soothe aching muscles:
2 drops Lemongrass,
4 drops Ginger, 4 drops Lavandin

To ease indigestion or stomach tension:
2 drops Lemongrass,
4 drops Coriander Seed,
4 drops Mandarin

105

Lavandin *(Lavandula × intermedia)*

A tough and vigorous shrub that thrives in the hot Mediterranean climate of southern France, lavandin is a cross between true lavender (see pp.134–5) and spike lavender (see pp.108–9). Its flowers are usually purple, although a white variety also exists. Taller than true lavender, with stronger stalks and larger flowerheads, lavandin also produces a higher yield of essential oil, and the oils have very different aromas: Lavandin essential oil is sharp, peppery, medicinal, fresh and uplifting, with sweeter notes as it evaporates; its effects are stimulating and energizing. True Lavender essential oil is softer, sweeter and more floral, and is well-known for its calming, relaxing and soothing effects.

Safety first

- Lavandin essential oil is non-toxic, non-irritating and non-sensitizing, so is safe for all skin types.
- Avoid using Lavandin if you suffer from epilepsy, as its high camphor content could cause seizures.

Plant features: Evergreen shrub with tall flowers

Part of plant used: Flowering tops

Oil produced in: France

Extraction method: Steam distillation

Special blends

Add these essential oils to 20ml/4 tsp carrier oil:

To warm and loosen muscles: 4 drops Lavandin, 4 drops Rosemary, 2 drops Ginger

To unblock respiratory passages: 4 drops Lavandin, 4 drops Myrtle, 2 drops Himalayan Cedarwood

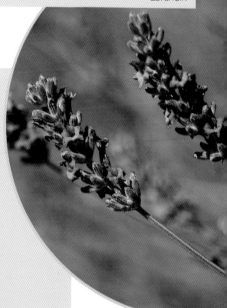

Supporting the spirit

- Lavandin expands the body's aura, making you feel freer.
- This oil strengthens your inner resolve to overcome obstacles.

Easing the mind

- To clear mental "fogginess", vaporize 2 drops Lavandin and 3 drops Spearmint.
- To relieve anxiety, place 2 drops Lavandin on a tissue and inhale.

Healing the body

- To warm cold limbs, ease muscular aches and improve circulation, mix Lavandin with Rosemary and Ginger in a carrier oil (see first blend, left) and apply to the affected areas.
- To loosen stiff muscles after sports, again apply Lavandin with Rosemary and Ginger in a carrier oil (again, see first blend, left).
- To ease breathing, mix Lavandin, Myrtle and Himalayan Cedarwood in a carrier oil (see second blend, left) and rub it into the chest.

Keywords
Energizing
Expansive
Clearing

107

Spike Lavender (*Lavandula latifolia*)

This hardy species of lavender boasts long, lance-shaped, grey-green leaves that are much larger than those of true lavender (see pp.134–5), plus tall, flowering spikes. Spike lavender grows wild in the southern Mediterranean, especially in Spain, Italy and France. Compared with true Lavender, the oil's aroma is sharper and more herbal, with strong camphor and woody notes. The 17th-century herbalist Nicholas Culpeper recommended spike lavender flowers for headaches and muscle pains. He also advised using the herb sparingly, as it has a powerful effect; the same is true of the oil.

Plant features: Evergreen shrub; blue-grey flowers	
Part of plant used: Flowering tops	
Oil produced in: Spain, Italy, France	
Extraction method: Steam distillation	

Safety first
- Spike Lavender essential oil is non-toxic, non-irritating and non-sensitizing, but use only a small amount.
- If you suffer from epilepsy, avoid Spike Lavender as its camphor content could cause seizures.

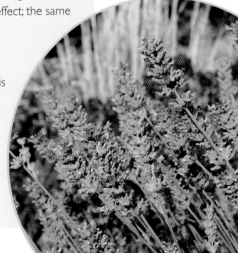

Supporting the spirit

- Spike Lavender will renew your connection to the wide-open spaces of Nature.
- This oil lightens the heart, giving courage to embrace the future and anything new.

Easing the mind

- To lift depression and renew hope, vaporize 2 drops Spike Lavender with 4 drops Lemon.
- To ease mental stress, vaporize 2 drops Spike Lavender with 4 drops Peppermint.

Healing the body

- To soothe aching muscles, and ease spasms and pain, mix Spike Lavender with Plai and Silver Fir in a carrier oil (see first blend, right) and apply it to the affected areas.
- To ease rheumatism, again apply Spike Lavender mixed with Plai and Silver Fir in a carrier oil (again, see first blend, right).
- To ease period pain and revive energy, mix Spike Lavender, Sweet Marjoram and Vetiver in a carrier oil (see second blend, right) and rub it into the lower abdomen.

Keywords
Opening
Freeing
Expansive

Special blends

Add these essential oils to 20ml/4 tsp carrier oil:

To warm muscles and ease rheumatic pain:
2 drops Spike Lavender, 4 drops Plai, 4 drops Silver Fir

To relieve painful periods:
2 drops Spike Lavender, 6 drops Sweet Marjoram, 2 drops Vetiver

109

Scots Pine *(Pinus sylvestris)*

Native to many northern latitudes, especially Scotland (hence its name), Russia, Scandinavia and Austria, this tall tree can grow to heights of up to 40m/130ft. It has deep fissures in its bark and pairs of long, stiff, dark-green needles, and it is these needles that yield the essential oil. Scots Pine essential oil is used extensively in the pharmaceutical industry to make liniments for sports injuries, as well as medicines for coughs and respiratory complaints. It has an invigoratingly fresh aroma, which is full of soft, fresh notes and woody hints. In perfumery, this oil is often used in fragrances for men.

Safety first
Scots Pine is non-toxic and non-irritating. However, do not use this essential oil if you have allergy-prone or sensitive skin.

Supporting the spirit
- Scots Pine will help to cleanse the spirit and clear away negativity, so is particularly useful if you are preparing for meditation.
- This oil helps you to cast off deep-held

Plant features:
Tall evergreen tree

Part of plant used:
Needles

Oil produced in: Scotland, Russia, Scandinavia, Austria

Extraction method:
Steam distillation

Special blends

Add these essential oils to 20ml/4 tsp carrier oil:

To encourage self-confidence:
2 drops Scots Pine,
4 drops Nutmeg,
4 drops Bergamot

To ease overworked muscles:
2 drops Scots Pine,
4 drops Spike Lavender,
4 drops Ginger

anxieties and open the door
to new solutions.

Easing the mind

- To ease nervous exhaustion
  through stress, take a bath with
  2 drops Scots Pine and 4 drops
  Orange Leaf.
- To boost confidence in your
  decisions and to help you to
  persevere, mix Scots Pine,
  Nutmeg and Bergamot in a carrier
  oil (see first blend, left) and rub the blend
  gently into any areas of tension.

Healing the body

- To help to relieve and relax painful, stiff
  muscles, mix Scots Pine with Spike Lavender
  and Ginger in a carrier oil (see second blend,
  left) and massage the blend into the affected
  areas as often you need to.
- To warm chilly limbs and ease physical
  tiredness, take a bath with 2 drops Scots
  Pine and 2 drops Cardamom.

Keywords
Fresh
Bracing
Invigorating

111

Rosemary *(Rosmarinus officinalis)*

Native to the arid seashores of the southern Mediterranean, where it still thrives, Rosemary is now cultivated all over the world. Its strong aroma is concentrated in its vibrant and vigorous green leaves, which are used as a popular culinary flavouring, as well as a healing herb. The Ancient Greeks burned branches of rosemary as incense, as its high content of essential oil makes a superbly fragrant smoke. Rosemary essential oil has a powerful effect, so always use moderate amounts. One of the most fresh and pungent oils, its aroma is instantly youthful and deliciously herbaceous.

Plant features:
Vigorous evergreen shrub

Part of plant used:
Leaves

Oil produced in:
Spain, Tunisia

Extraction method:
Steam distillation

Safety first

- Rosemary oil is non-toxic, non-irritating and non-sensitizing, so is safe for all skin types.
- Avoid Rosemary if you suffer from epilepsy, as its high camphor content could cause seizures.
- Do not use this powerful oil during pregnancy.

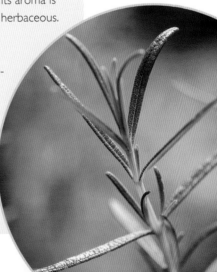

Supporting the spirit

- Rosemary will awaken the fire of creativity in your heart, encouraging inspiration.
- This oil will fire your passion for life and give you the vision to follow your path bravely.

Easing the mind

- To overcome sluggishness and revive mental clarity, mix Rosemary with Peppermint and Grapefruit in a carrier oil (see first blend, right) and rub it into the neck and shoulders.
- To clear mental fatigue and renew enthusiasm for your work, vaporize 3 drops Rosemary and 3 drops Lemon.

Healing the body

- To stimulate and warm sore muscles, especially before or after playing sports, mix Rosemary with Black Pepper and Vetiver in a carrier oil (see second blend, right) and massage it into the relevant areas.
- To ease chronic backache, take a warm bath containing 2 drops Rosemary and 4 drops Lavender.

Keywords

Vibrant

Invigorating

Strengthening

Special blends

Add these essential oils to 20ml/4 tsp carrier oil:

To bring back zest to a tired mind:
4 drops Rosemary,
2 drops Peppermint,
4 drops Grapefruit

To revitalize aching muscles:
4 drops Rosemary,
4 drops Black Pepper,
2 drops Vetiver

113

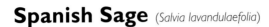

Spanish Sage (*Salvia lavandulaefolia*)

This special kind of sage from Spain is unique because its leaves smell more like lavender than sage – hence its botanical name *lavandulaefolia*, which means "with leaves like lavender". The overall aroma of this herb is highly unusual: it is fresh, camphoraceous and slightly pungent, with definite sweet floral notes in the background – and the essential oil is the same. Several types of sage are used throughout Europe in herbal medicine, as well as being available as essential oils. They include common sage (but this oil is too strong to use in aromatherapy); clary sage (see pp.206–7); and, this one, Spanish sage. All sages – in both herb and essential-oil forms – are regarded as strengthening and revitalizing, with powerful effects on body and mind. They should all be used in moderation.

Safety first

- Spanish sage is non-toxic, non-sensitizing and non-irritant, so is safe for all skin types.
- Avoid this oil if you suffer from epilepsy as its high camphor content could cause seizures.
- Do not use Spanish Sage during pregnancy.

Plant features;
Aromatic evergreen shrub

Part of plant used:
Leaves

Oil produced in:
Spain

Extraction method:
Steam distillation

Special blends

Add these essential oils to 20ml/4 tsp carrier oil:

To loosen muscular stiffness:
4 drops Spanish Sage, 2 drops Ginger, 4 drops Rosemary

To boost immunity during viruses:
4 drops Spanish Sage, 4 drops Manuka, 2 drops Black Pepper

Supporting the spirit
- Spanish Sage revives the emotions, aiding recovery from disappointment or sadness.
- This oil encourages faith in yourself and generates the energy to move forward in life.

Easing the mind
- To lift depression and ease anxiety, take a bath with 2 drops Spanish Sage and 4 drops Orange Leaf.
- To unravel confused thoughts and enable fresh, clear thinking, vaporize 2 drops Spanish Sage and 4 drops Myrtle.

Healing the body
- To ease out stiff, painful muscles, mix Spanish Sage with Ginger and Rosemary in a carrier oil (see first blend, left) and massage it into the sore areas.
- To support the immune system during colds or flu, mix Spanish Sage with Manuka and Black Pepper in a carrier oil (see second blend, left) and apply it in a chest massage, morning and evening.

Keywords
Refreshing
Revitalizing
Enlivening

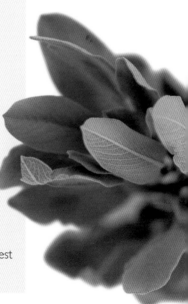

Vetiver *(Vetiveria zizanoides)*

In India and Nepal, vetiver is planted to protect hillsides from erosion during the monsoon. The grass's tangled root system holds the soil together and is also the part of the plant that yields Vetiver essential oil. This oil is thick and dark brown, with an aroma of deepest earth, and woody and smoky undertones. In blends, use Vetiver in only small amounts; otherwise its aroma takes over – it adds deep, rich aromatic notes to any combination. In Sri Lanka and India, Vetiver is known as the "oil of tranquillity" because of its deeply calming effect.

Plant features:
Tough, aromatic grass

Part of plant used:
Roots

Oil produced in:
India, Indonesia, Sri Lanka

Extraction method:
Steam distillation

Safety first
Vetiver essential oil is non-toxic, non-irritating and non-sensitizing, so is safe for all skin types.

Supporting the spirit
• Vetiver deepens spiritual connection to the Earth, the source of our strength.
• This oil grounds spiritual awareness in the body.

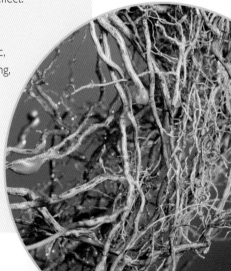

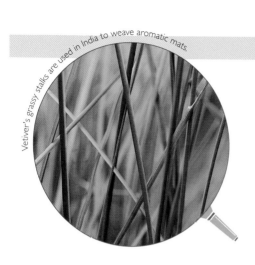

Vetiver's grassy stalks are used in India to weave aromatic mats.

Keywords

Earthy

Grounding

Warming

Easing the mind

- To relieve insomnia, take a bath containing 2 drops Vetiver and 4 drops Australian Sandalwood just before bed.
- To soothe mental exhaustion, mix Vetiver with Neroli and Linaloe Wood in a carrier oil (see first blend, right) and stroke it into your body.

Healing the body

- To release the physical effects of emotional stress, rub a blend of Vetiver, Cardamom and Sweet Orange in a carrier oil (see second blend, right) into the areas of most tension.
- To ease rheumatism and stiff joints, take a bath with 2 drops Vetiver and 4 drops Plai.

Special blends

Add these essential oils to 20ml/4 tsp carrier oil:

To care for a depleted mind and encourage proper rest:
2 drops Vetiver, 4 drops Neroli, 4 drops Linaloe Wood

To penetrate the muscles and ease physical tension:
2 drops Vetiver, 4 drops Cardamom, 4 drops Sweet Orange

Plai (*Zingiber montanum*)

Closely related to ginger (see pp. 120–21), plai has a thick root with bright orange-coloured flesh. In its native Thailand, the fresh root is highly valued as a traditional medicine – hot poultices made with freshly chopped, steamed root are applied directly to chronic backache and to osteoarthritic joints to relieve pain and inflammation. Thai herbal medicine also uses plai to treat acne, sun-spots or scars, while a lotion made by soaking the root in vegetable oil is used to massage women recovering from childbirth. In aromatherapy, Plai essential oil is a successful pain-reliever and anti-inflammatory. Its aroma is soft and sweet, with a hint of spice.

Safety first

Plai essential oil is non-toxic, non-irritating and non-sensitizing, so is safe for all skin types.

Supporting the spirit

- This essential oil will give you the inner strength to cope with life's major events.
- Plai helps to build self-confidence, inner resilience and the strength to persevere.

Plant features: Tropical plant with fleshy root

Part of plant used: Roots

Oil produced in: Thailand

Extraction method: Steam distillation

Special blends

Add these essential oils to 20ml/4 tsp carrier oil:

To ease discomfort and swelling:
4 drops Plai, 4 drops German Chamomile, 2 drops Yarrow

To relieve abdominal cramping:
4 drops Plai, 4 drops Sweet Marjoram, 2 drops Lavender

Easing the mind

- To soothe mental stress and release worry, bathe with 4 drops Plai and 2 drops Neroli.
- To dissolve away chronic mental exhaustion, encouraging the mind to let go, vaporize 2 drops Plai and 4 drops Tangerine.

Healing the body

- To relieve pain and stiffness in osteoarthritic joints, sports injuries or pulled muscles, mix Plai with German Chamomile and Yarrow in a carrier oil (see first blend, left) and rub it into the affected areas.
- To soothe the inflammation of rheumatoid arthritis, take a warm bath with 4 drops Plai and 2 drops Yarrow.
- To ease stomach cramps or period pain, massage the lower abdomen with a blend of Plai, Sweet Marjoram and Lavender in a carrier oil (see second blend, left), then rest with a hot-water bottle over the area.

Keywords
Soothing
Stabilizing
Nurturing

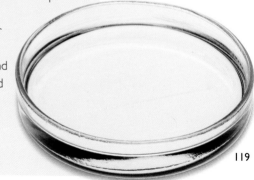

119

Ginger *(Zingiber officinalis)*

One of the most important spices in China and India, ginger provides a digestive stimulant in the cuisine of both nations. In addition, in their traditional medicines, ginger is used remedially to treat all kinds of conditions, including colds, coughs, flu, rheumatism, aching muscles and joints, and even malaria. Fresh ginger is very warming and helps to fight viral infections by slightly raising body temperature, which makes it harder for viruses to survive. Ginger essential oil has a different aroma to the pungency of fresh ginger root – the oil is softer and sweeter, with a very pleasant, spicy fragrance.

Safety first
- Ginger is non-toxic and non-irritant.
- This oil is mildly sensitizing: avoid using it if you have sensitive or allergy-prone skin.

Supporting the spirit
- Ginger essential oil stimulates optimism and boosts your initiative to take action.
- Ginger revitalizes self-confidence, giving you the energy to move forward in life.

Plant features: Tropical flower with elegant leaves

Part of plant used: Roots

Oil produced in: China, India

Extraction method: Steam distillation

Special blends

Add these essential oils to 20ml/4 tsp carrier oil:

To increase blood-flow to cold limbs:
2 drops Ginger, 4 drops Black Pepper, 4 drops Cardamom

To relieve digestive problems:
2 drops Ginger, 4 drops Spearmint, 4 drops Sweet Orange

Easing the mind

- To ease anxiety and renew vitality, vaporize 2 drops Ginger and 4 drops Sweet Orange.
- To transform listlessness and apathy into focus and inspiration, take a bath with 2 drops Ginger and 3 drops Cardamom.

Healing the body

- To warm chilly limbs and to ease stiffness, mix Ginger with Black Pepper and Cardamom in a carrier oil (see first blend, left) and apply it using vigorous strokes to the parts of your body that feel cold and/or stiff.
- To relieve muscular cramps, spasms and aches, take a bath with 2 drops Ginger and 4 drops Coriander Seed.
- To ease digestive cramping, indigestion or wind, blend Ginger, Spearmint and Sweet Orange in a carrier oil (see second blend, left) and massage it, clockwise, into the abdomen.
- To relieve morning or travel sickness, place 2 drops Ginger on a tissue and inhale.

Keywords

Comforting

Warming

Strengthening

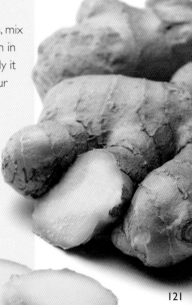

121

Yarrow (*Achillea millefolium*)

Often dismissed as a weed, this humble-looking plant has been valued as a supreme wound-healer since the Dark Ages. The essential oil contains the anti-inflammatory azulene. Yarrow's unusual aroma is sharp and very sweet, with slight camphor and wood notes.

Plant features:
Greyish-green herb with white flowers

Part of plant used:
Leaves and flowers

Oil produced in:
Hungary, Germany

Extraction method:
Steam distillation

Safety first
• Yarrow oil is non-toxic and non-irritating.
• Avoid this oil if you have allergy-prone skin.
• Avoid this oil if you suffer from epilepsy.
• Do not use Yarrow oil if you are pregnant.

Supporting the spirit
• Yarrow essential oil will help you to develop a sense of inner peace and tranquillity.
• Yarrow can heal a spirit wounded by anger.

Easing the mind
• To cool emotions, take a bath with 2 drops Yarrow and 4 drops Neroli.

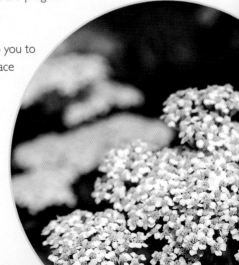

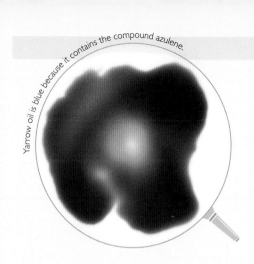

Yarrow oil is blue because it contains the compound azulene.

Keywords

Cooling

Protective

Nurturing

• To dissolve emotional blockages, mix Yarrow with Rose Otto and Mandarin in a carrier oil (see first blend, right) and apply it gently.

Healing the body

• To soothe eczema, dermatitis, itching or irritation, mix Yarrow, Roman Chamomile and Palmarosa in a carrier oil (see second blend, right) and apply it to the affected areas.

• To heal deep cuts, apply 4 drops Yarrow, 2 drops Tea Tree and 4 drops Myrrh in 20g/4 tsp Skin Mousse (see pp.42–3).

• To soothe inflammation caused by sprains or pulled muscles, use a cold compress with 4 drops Yarrow.

Special blends

Add these essential oils to 20ml/4 tsp carrier oil:

To enable you to release your emotions:
2 drops Yarrow, 4 drops Rose Otto, 4 drops Mandarin

To soothe sore or itching skin:
4 drops Yarrow, 2 drops Roman Chamomile, 4 drops Palmarosa

Roman Chamomile (*Anthemis nobilis*)

The name "chamomile" comes from two Greek words – *chamai* meaning "on the ground" and *melon* meaning "apple", and this low-growing herb has a wonderful apple-like scent all around it. Roman chamomile's flowers are large in contrast to German chamomile (see pp.136–7), but the flowers of both species are soothing to the skin, as well as the digestive and nervous systems. Roman Chamomile essential oil has a pale, blue-green colour, as it contains a small amount of azulene – a blue anti-inflammatory constituent. Fresh and soft-smelling, the oil retains the plant's apple-like notes.

Safety first
- This oil is non-toxic and non-irritating.
- Roman Chamomile oil is a mild sensitizer: avoid it if you have allergy-prone skin.

Supporting the spirit
- Roman Chamomile promotes a sense of innocence and child-like spontaneity.
- This essential oil will enable the simple expression of your personal truth.

Plant features: Herb with feathery foliage and daisy-like flowers

Part of plant used: Flowers

Oil produced in: UK, Hungary

Extraction method: Steam distillation

Special blends

Add these essential oils to 20ml/4 tsp carrier oil:

To soothe irritated skin: 4 drops Roman Chamomile, 4 drops Neroli, 2 drops Lavender.

To relax and ease backache in pregnancy (only after 6 months): 2 drops Roman Chamomile, 2 drops Australian Sandalwood

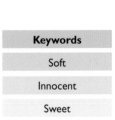

Easing the mind

- To ease away stress, vaporize 3 drops Roman Chamomile and 2 drops Sweet Orange.
- To quieten internal chatter and ease insomnia, take a bath with 4 drops Roman Chamomile and 2 drops Australian Sandalwood.

Healing the body

- To heal inflamed skin or eczema, apply to the affected areas a blend of Roman Chamomile, Neroli and Lavender, in a base of either 20g/4 tsp Skin Mousse (see pp.42–3) or 20ml/4 tsp carrier oil (see first blend, left).
- To ease sore skin on a baby, try 1 drop Roman Chamomile in 20g/4 tsp Skin Mousse (see pp.42–3).
- To relieve backache in late pregnancy, apply Roman Chamomile and Australian Sandalwood in a carrier oil (see second blend, left), using gentle massage.
- To relieve sprains, use a cold compress with 4 drops Roman Chamomile.

Keywords
Soft
Innocent
Sweet

125

Frankincense (*Boswellia carterii*)

Originating from the arid climates of North Africa and Oman, Frankincense essential oil begins life as a resin that oozes out of damaged bark. The Ancient Egyptians used this resin as incense, a preservative in the embalming process, a perfume, a cosmetic ingredient and an offering to the gods. The essential oil retains all the warm, pungent, sweet notes of the resin from which it is extracted. It is one of the most important oils for skincare, with remarkable rejuvenating and healing properties.

Plant features: Tall shrub with papery bark

Part of plant used: Resin

Oil produced in: Somalia, Oman

Extraction method: Steam distillation

Safety first

Frankincense is non-toxic, non-irritating and non-sensitizing, so is safe for all skin types.

Supporting the spirit

- Frankincense brings peace and balance, encouraging a meditative state.
- This essential oil clears your awareness as you deepen your spiritual understanding.

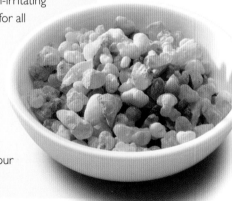

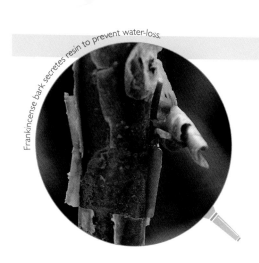
Frankincense bark secretes resin to prevent water-loss.

Keywords

Rejuvenating

Meditative

Harmonizing

Easing the mind
- To raise low self-esteem, vaporize 3 drops Frankincense and 3 drops Cardamom.
- To calm anxiety, take a bath with 2 drops Frankincense and 4 drops Rose Geranium.

Healing the body
- To improve skin-tone, mix Frankincense, Rose Otto and Neroli in a carrier (see first blend, right) and massage into the face nightly.
- To heal cuts and grazes, mix Frankincense with Myrrh and Manuka in a carrier oil (see second blend, right) and apply to the wound.
- To heal infected skin, use a hot compress with 4 drops Frankincense and 2 drops Tea Tree.

Special blends

Add these essential oils to 20ml/4 tsp carrier oil:

To rejuvenate mature skin:
4 drops Frankincense,
2 drops Rose Otto,
4 drops Neroli

To heal wounds:
4 drops Frankincense,
2 drops Myrrh, 4 drops Manuka

127

Elemi *(Canarium luzonicum)*

Native to the Philippine Islands, the elemi tree is a member of the same botanical family as Frankincense (see pp.126–7) and Myrrh (see pp.150–51). All these trees produce gums that have been used since ancient times for healing and as incense. Elemi essential oil is extracted from the gum and has a beautiful fragrance – it is fresh, spicy and slightly citrusy, with wonderful warm, resiny undertones. Although it is unusual and available only from specialist essential-oil suppliers, Elemi is one of the most effective oils for treating skin problems, such as acne or wounds that are slow to heal.

Safety first
Elemi essential oil is non-toxic, non-irritating and non-sensitizing, making it suitable to use on all skin types.

Supporting the spirit
- Elemi esssential oil eases a heavy heart, lightening emotional burdens.
- This oil brings a sense of deep peace and inner contentment to the spirit.

Plant features: Tropical tree with lush foliage

Part of plant used: Gum

Oil produced in: Philippines

Extraction method: Steam distillation

Special blends

Add these essential oils to 20ml/4 tsp carrier oil:

To restore dry skin:
4 drops Elemi, 2 drops Rose Absolute, 4 drops Frankincense

To smooth out wrinkles:
4 drops Elemi, 2 drops Neroli, 4 drops Palmarosa

Easing the mind

- To calm emotional anxiety, take a bath with 2 drops Elemi and 4 drops Grapefruit.
- To lift depression and relieve feelings of low self-worth, vaporize 3 drops Elemi and 3 drops Frankincense.

Healing the body

- To heal deep cuts, especially if they are slow to recover, apply 4 drops Elemi, 2 drops Tea Tree and 4 drops Myrrh in 20g/4 tsp Skin Mousse (see pp.42–3) to the affected area.
- To strengthen and rejuvenate dry skin, mix Elemi with Rose Absolute and Frankincense in a carrier oil (see first blend, left) and massage it in daily where your skin needs it most.
- To replenish mature skin, apply a nightly treatment of Elemi with Neroli and Palmarosa in a carrier oil (see second blend, left) to your face.

Keywords

Opening

Light

Restoring

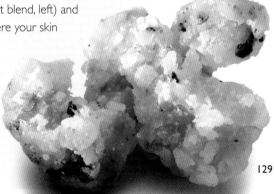

129

Orange Leaf (*Citrus aurantium*)

Also known as Petitgrain, Orange Leaf essential oil is obtained from the aromatic leaves of the bitter orange tree, the flowers of which produce Neroli (Orange Blossom essential oil; see pp.256–7). The tree was originally native to China, although nowadays it also thrives in the hot climates of southern France, and of Algeria, Spain and Paraguay. The leaves are speckled with tiny sacs of essential oil that you can see clearly if you hold a leaf up to the light. The oil has a wonderful youthful, fresh, sweet and slightly woody aroma. It nourishes combination or oily skin, leaving behind a lovely citrusy scent.

Safety first
This essential oil is non-toxic, non-irritating and non-sensitizing, so is safe for all skin types.

Supporting the spirit
• Orange Leaf fosters a positive attitude to challenges, helping you to find solutions.
• This oil generates feelings of joy and hopefulness in the spirit.

Plant features: Evergreen tree with wrinkled, bitter orange fruit

Part of plant used: Leaves

Oil produced in: France, Algeria, Spain, Paraguay

Extraction method: Steam distillation

Special blends

Add these essential oils to 20ml/4 tsp carrier oil:

To calm emotional stress:
4 drops Orange Leaf, 2 drops Neroli, 4 drops Sweet Orange

To tone oily or combination skin:
4 drops Orange Leaf, 2 drops Ylang Ylang, 4 drops Australian Sandalwood

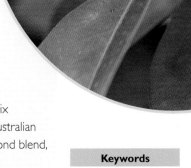

Easing the mind

- To soothe overwrought emotions, use a blend of Orange Leaf, Neroli and Sweet Orange in a carrier oil (see first blend, left) and massage it gently into areas of tension.
- To relieve nervous exhaustion and lift depression, take a bath with 4 drops Orange Leaf and 2 drops Neroli.

Healing the body

- To clear oily or combination skins, mix Orange Leaf with Ylang Ylang and Australian Sandalwood in a carrier oil (see second blend, left) and apply it to your face nightly.
- To balance sensitive skin on the face, apply a mixture of 2 drops Orange Leaf and 2 drops Geranium in 20g/4 tsp Skin Mousse (see pp.42–3) every night before bed.
- To ease physical tiredness in late pregnancy (after 6 months), take a bath with 2 drops Orange Leaf and 2 drops Lavender.

Keywords
Uplifting
Refreshing
Balancing

131

Bergamot (*Citrus bergamia*)

Produced in the area around Bergamo, in northern Italy (hence its name), bergamot is a type of bitter orange with greenish-yellow skin. Its pulp is too sour to eat, so the fruit is produced solely for the extraction of essential oil from the peel. It is not possible to grow bergamot trees from seed. Young shoots are grafted onto rootstock of other citrus species, such as bitter orange or lemon, to propagate new trees. Bergamot oil was an ingredient in the earliest formula of "eau de Cologne", in the 18th century. This oil has a delightful aroma: fresh and young with strong citrus notes, and a sweetness as it evaporates.

Plant features: Citrus tree grafted on rootstock

Part of plant used: Fruit peel

Oil produced in: Italy

Extraction method: Expression

Safety first
- Bergamot is phototoxic: avoid massaging it into your skin if you are going out into strong sunlight.
- This oil is non-toxic, non-irritating and non-sensitizing, so is safe for all skin types.

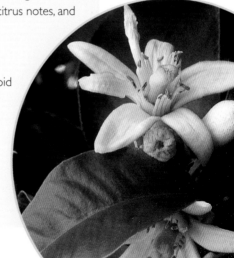

Supporting the spirit

- Bergamot essential oil gently releases pent-up emotions, enabling you to express your feelings effectively but realistically.
- This oil relieves feelings of apathy and listlessness.

Easing the mind

- To ease severe emotional anxiety, take a bath with 2 drops Bergamot and 4 drops Neroli.
- To ease and calm grief, mix Bergamot with Rose Otto and Australian Sandalwood in a carrier oil (see first blend, right) and apply it to your body in long, soothing strokes.

Healing the body

- To clear and cleanse oily or problem skin, or acne, mix Bergamot with Sweet Orange and Linaloe Wood in a carrier oil (see second blend, right) and apply it to your face, or any other problem areas, as necessary.
- To cleanse and heal infected cuts or boils, use a hot compress with 2 drops Bergamot and 4 drops Tea Tree.

Keywords

Refreshing

Euphoric

Nurturing

Special blends

Add these essential oils to 20ml/4 tsp carrier oil:

To soothe the pain of grief or loss:
2 drops Bergamot,
4 drops Rose Otto,
4 drops Australian Sandalwood

To clear oily or problem skin:
2 drops Bergamot,
4 drops Sweet Orange,
4 drops Linaloe Wood

133

Lavender *(Lavandula angustifolia)*

Originally native to the region of the southern Mediterranean, lavender is now found in much of western Europe. The essential oil has a refreshing aroma: the stems and leaves give camphoraceous notes that are softened by floral sweetness from the flowers.

Plant features:
Shrub with purple flowers

Part of plant used:
Flowering stalks

Oil produced in:
UK, France, Bulgaria

Extraction method:
Steam distillation

Safety first
Lavender is non-toxic, non-irritating and non-sensitizing, so is safe for all skin types.

Supporting the spirit
• This oil brings deep relaxation.
• Lavender encourages compassion and gentleness toward others.

Easing the mind
• To calm emotional anxiety, take a bath with 2 drops Lavender and 2 drops Linaloe Wood.
• To help to relieve insomnia, vaporize 4 drops Lavender and 2 drops Sweet Orange.

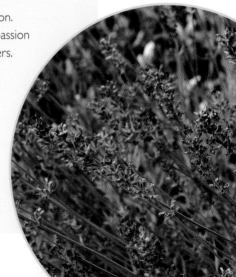

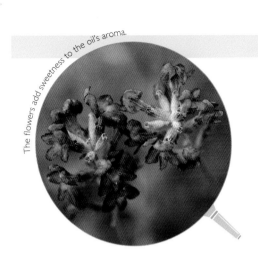

The flowers add sweetness to the oil's aroma.

Soothing

Calming

Reassuring

Healing the body

- To heal burns, sunburn or eczema, apply a blend of Lavender, Roman Chamomile and Spearmint in a carrier (see first blend, right).
- To calm irritated baby skin, massage in a blend of 1 drop Lavender in 20ml/4 tsp carrier oil.
- To relieve muscular aches, take a bath with 4 drops Lavender and 2 drops Vetiver.
- To ease backache during late pregnancy, mix Lavender and Linaloe Wood in a carrier oil (see second blend, right) and apply it to your back using gentle massage.
- To relieve painful swelling resulting from a sprain, use a cold compress with 4 drops Lavender and 2 drops Yarrow.

Special blends

Add these essential oils to 20ml/4 tsp carrier oil:

To soothe burns or sunburn:
6 drops Lavender, 2 drops Roman Chamomile, 2 drops Spearmint (you could use 20g/4 tsp Skin Mousse – see pp.42–3 – rather than a carrier)

To ease backache in pregnancy (only after 6 months):
2 drops Lavender, 2 drops Linaloe Wood

135

German Chamomile (*Matricaria recutita*)

The German chamomile plant is commonly used to make a herbal tea that helps to relieve nervous complaints and digestive problems. The plant's essential oil is made by picking its daisy-like flowers as they start to bloom, then drying them to preserve the active ingredients and distilling them. One of the most important oils for treating skin problems, German Chamomile contains azulene, an anti-inflammatory that gives the oil a deep blue colour. The oil's aroma is medicinal, with bittersweet notes.

Plant features: Herb with feathery foliage and small daisy-like flowers

Part of plant used:
Dried flowers

Oil produced in:
Hungary

Extraction method:
Steam distillation

Safety first

German Chamomile is non-toxic, non-irritating and non-sensitizing, so is safe for all skin types.

Supporting the spirit

- German Chamomile essential oil cools emotional over-excitement.
- This oil grounds and centres the spirit, creating a deep sense of inner calm.

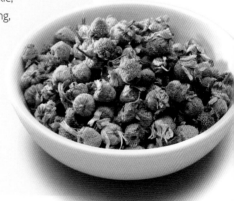

Easing the mind

- To ease mental and emotional stress, take a bath with 1 drop German Chamomile and 4 drops Lavender.
- To calm extreme nervous tension, mix German Chamomile with Linaloe Wood and Lavender in a carrier oil (see first blend, right) and rub it into areas of tension in your body.

Healing the body

- To soothe eczema, psoriasis or burned skin, apply a balm of 2 drops German Chamomile, 6 drops Lavender and 2 drops Frankincense in 20g/4 tsp Skin Mousse (see pp.42–3).
- To nourish sensitive skin on the face, apply a nightly mix of German Chamomile and Rose Absolute in a carrier (see second blend, right).
- To ease stiff or painful muscles and joints, take a bath with 2 drops German Chamomile and 2 drops Vetiver.
- To reduce inflammation caused by sprains, pulled muscles or other such injuries, use a cold compress with 2 drops German Chamomile and 2 drops Peppermint.

Keywords

Powerful

Strengthening

Soothing

Special blends

Add these essential oils to 20ml/4 tsp carrier oil:

To relieve physical tension caused by anxiety:
2 drops German Chamomile, 4 drops Linaloe Wood, 4 drops Lavender

To fortify sensitive skin:
1 drop German Chamomile, 3 drops Rose Absolute (note the low concentration)

137

Tea Tree (*Melaleuca alternifolia*)

Native to Australia, the tea tree produces one of the most well-known essential oils. The tree was first discovered by Captain Cook's sailors in the 18th century – they brewed a tea with its leaves to fight scurvy, hence the plant's common name. The indigenous Aborigines were already well aware of the healing powers of the leaves, using them to relieve respiratory problems and headaches. Research has proved that Tea Tree essential oil has powerful antimicrobial and antifungal effects. Its aroma is fresh, pungent and medicinal, with sweeter woody notes as it evaporates.

Safety first
- Tea Tree is non-toxic and non-irritant.
- This oil is a mild sensitizer: avoid it if you have sensitive or allergy-prone skin.
- This oil goes off quickly; keep it no longer than six months, or one year in the refrigerator.

Supporting the spirit
- This oil restores feelings of optimism.
- Tea Tree oil renews energy levels.

Plant features: Vigorous evergreen tree

Part of plant used: Leaves

Oil produced in: Australia

Extraction method: Steam distillation

Special blends

Add these essential oils to 20ml/4 tsp carrier oil:

To clear acne, oily or combination skin:
4 drops Tea Tree,
4 drops Lemon,
4 drops Geranium

To boost immunity against viruses:
4 drops Tea Tree, 2 drops Black Pepper, 4 drops Bergamot

Easing the mind

- To refresh thought processes, vaporize 3 drops Tea Tree and 3 drops Peppermint.
- To restore self-confidence, take a bath with 2 drops Tea Tree and 4 drops Tangerine.

Healing the body

- To speed the healing of infected cuts, wounds and insect bites, place 2 drops Tea Tree on a cotton bud and apply the oil neat to the affected area.
- To heal acne and clarify oily or combination skin, mix Tea Tree with Lemon and Geranium in a carrier oil (see first blend, left) and apply it to your face, or other affected areas, nightly.
- To fight viral infections, such as flu, mix Tea Tree with Black Pepper and Bergamot in a carrier oil (see second blend, left) and massage the blend into the chest twice a day.
- To draw out and speed the healing of a skin infection, apply a hot compress with 2 drops Tea Tree and 2 drops Bergamot.

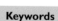

Keywords

Bracing

Youthful

Powerful

Moroccan Chamomile *(Ormenis mixta)*

This essential oil comes from a species of wild flower native to Morocco. Although the flower looks like chamomile and has that common name, botanically this plant has totally different biochemistry to the true chamomiles (Roman and German; see pp. 124–5 and 136–7). Sometimes called Ormenis oil, Moroccan Chamomile essential oil is dark yellow, whereas true chamomiles, which contain the compound azulene, are blue. It has a very different aroma, too – it is fresh and herbaceous with light medicinal notes. Moroccan Chamomile helps to boost liver function, and soothes both the skin and the nervous system.

Safety first
There have been no reports of safety issues associated with using Moroccan Chamomile.

Supporting the spirit
• Moroccan Chamomile soothes fiery emotions to bring a sense of inner stability.
• This oil "switches off" overactive thought patterns to enable deep inner quiet.

Plant features: Wild flower with daisy-like blooms

Part of plant used: Flowers

Oil produced in: Morocco

Extraction method: Steam distillation

Special blends

Add these essential oils to 20ml/4 tsp carrier oil:

To balance oily or combination skin:
2 drops Moroccan Chamomile, 4 drops Mandarin, 4 drops Geranium

To relieve physical exhaustion:
4 drops Moroccan Chamomile, 4 drops Lavender, 2 drops Neroli

Easing the mind
- To soothe away depression and anxiety, take a bath with 2 drops Moroccan Chamomile and 4 drops Lavender.
- To ease the pressure when the mind is overloaded, vaporize 2 drops Moroccan Chamomile and 4 drops Sweet Orange.

Healing the body
- To clarify oily or combination skin, mix Moroccan Chamomile with Mandarin and Geranium in a carrier oil (see first blend, left) and apply it to your face nightly.
- To ease physical tiredness resulting from mental stress, mix Moroccan Chamomile with Lavender and Neroli in a carrier oil (see second blend, left) and rub it soothingly into areas where you feel you store tension.
- To help to ease menstrual pain, take a bath with 2 drops Moroccan Chamomile and 4 drops Sweet Marjoram.

Keywords
Fresh
Soft
Soothing

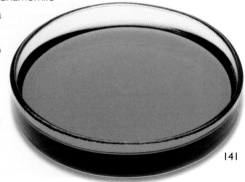

141

Geranium (*Pelargonium graveolens*)

There are more than 200 species of geranium, some scented and some not. The well-known essential oil is extracted from the leaves of a tropical, scented species originating from the island of Réunion in the Indian Ocean. On the surface of each leaf are thousands of tiny, silky hairs, and at the end of each hair is a minute sac filled with essential oil. Although Geranium oil is now available from elsewhere, the finest – which has a soft, richly sweet aroma – is still produced on Réunion.

Plant features: Tropical scented flower

Parts of plant used: Leaves

Oil produced in: Réunion

Extraction method: Steam distillation

Safety first

Geranium essential oil is non-toxic, non-irritating and non-sensitizing, so is safe for all skin types.

Supporting the spirit

- Geranium essential oil nurtures and soothes the "inner child", promoting a sense of inner peace.
- This oil lifts the spirit and soothes away stress.

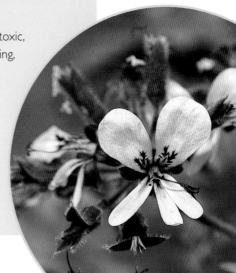

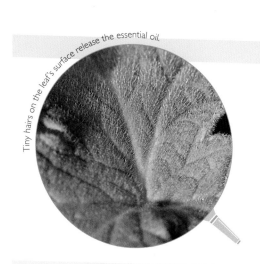

Tiny hairs on the leaf's surface release the essential oil.

Keywords

Balancing

Soft

Nurturing

Easing the mind

- To calm irritability, take a bath with 4 drops Geranium and 2 drops Mandarin.
- To relax the mind and ease insomnia, vaporize 3 drops Geranium and 3 drops Lavender in your bedroom before you go to sleep.

Healing the body

- To help to even out oily or combination skin, mix Geranium with Neroli and Roman Chamomile in a carrier oil (see first blend, right) and apply it to your face nightly.
- To nourish dry or mature skin, use a nighttime face blend of Geranium, Frankincense and Australian Sandalwood in a carrier oil (see second blend, right).

Special blends

Add these essential oils to 20ml/4 tsp carrier oil:

To soothe and balance oily or combination skin: 2 drops Geranium, 4 drops Neroli, 4 drops Roman Chamomile

To rehydrate dry skin: 4 drops Geranium, 4 drops Frankincense, 2 drops Australian Sandalwood

143

Rose Geranium *(Pelargonium roseum)*

Native to South Africa, the original home of all geranium species, this scented geranium has large, pink flowers with slightly serrated edges. Rose Geranium essential oil has a very sweet and soft, rosy aroma (it is much less sharp than the more common Geranium essential oil; see pp.142–3). The rose-like scent is why this oil is often used in perfumery as a substitute for Rose Otto (see pp.268–9), which is much more costly to produce. In aromatherapy, the rich, gentle fragrance of Rose Geranium is valued for a host of female-related issues, including to nurture and support the hormone cycles.

Safety first

Rose Geranium is non-toxic, non-irritant and non-sensitizing, so is safe for all skin types.

Supporting the spirit

- Rose Geranium nurtures and rejuvenates the inner feminine, boosting your sense of intuition, receptivity and openness.
- This oil encourages creativity and the expression of inner beauty.

Plant features: Scented geranium with large pink flowers

Part of plant used: Leaves and flowers

Oil produced in: South Africa

Extraction method: Steam distillation

Special blends

Add these essential oils to 20ml/4 tsp carrier oil:

To centre the emotions:
4 drops Rose Geranium,
2 drops Ylang Ylang,
4 drops Sweet Orange

To smooth out the appearance of dry skin:
2 drops Rose Geranium,
4 drops Palmarosa,
4 drops Linaloe Wood

Easing the mind

- To even out mood swings and ease mental stress, take a bath with 2 drops Rose Geranium and 4 drops Tangerine.
- To calm frustration and bring emotional stability, mix Rose Geranium with Ylang Ylang and Sweet Orange in a carrier oil (see first blend, left) and apply it gently to the areas where you store tension.

Healing the body

- To hydrate dry, wrinkled or mature skin, mix Rose Geranium with Palmarosa and Linaloe Wood in a carrier oil (see second blend, left) and apply it to your face using your fingertips.
- To ease the symptoms of PMS, such as fluid retention and tiredness, bathe with 2 drops Rose Geranium and 2 drops Clary Sage.
- To balance the hormones during the peri-menopause and the menopause, take a bath with 2 drops Rose Geranium, 1 drop Agnus Castus and 1 drop Neroli.

Keywords

Enveloping

Loving

Gentle

145

Patchouli (*Pogestemon cablin*)

The exotic fragrance of Patchouli oil instantly transports you to faraway lands – India, Indonesia and the Philippines, where the oil has been valued for centuries as a perfume. The leaves of the patchouli bush are covered with tiny hairs, each carrying a microscopic globule of essential oil. If you stroke the leaf's surface, you will therefore release tiny amounts of the thick, dark-brown oil onto your fingers. The aroma of Patchouli essential oil is deep, earthy and sensual. It is also very powerful, so you need use only small amounts when making up blends. Nevertheless, Patchouli adds amazing richness to any aromatherapy treatment.

Plant features: Shrub with pale green, velvety leaves

Part of plant used: Leaves

Oil produced in: India, Indonesia, Philippines

Extraction method: Steam distillation

Safety first
Patchouli is non-toxic, non-irritating and non-sensitizing, so is safe for all skin types.

Supporting the spirit
• Patchouli essential oil helps to build a balanced connection between body, mind and spirit.

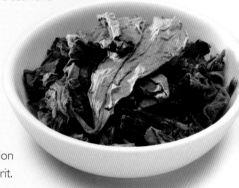

146

• This oil grounds and centres spiritual awareness in the body.

Easing the mind
• To soothe nervous exhaustion and deep emotional stress, take a bath with 2 drops Patchouli and 4 drops Neroli.
• To raise low sexual energy and overcome emotional vulnerability, mix Patchouli with Rose Absolute and Sweet Orange in a carrier oil (see first blend, right) and apply it to areas of tension; or ask a partner to apply it in a relaxing back massage.

Healing the body
• To hydrate and nourish dry, wrinkled or mature skin, mix Patchouli with Jasmine Absolute and Palmarosa (see second blend, right) and apply it to your face nightly, concentrating on the worst-affected areas.
• To heal acne, eczema or damaged skin, add 2 drops Patchouli, 4 drops Myrrh and 4 drops Frankincense to 20g/4 tsp Skin Mousse (see pp.42–3) and apply it to the affected areas.

| **Keywords** |
| Opening |
| Grounding |
| Mysterious |

| Special blends |

Add these essential oils to 20ml/4 tsp carrier oil:

To increase sexual energy and encourage emotional confidence:
2 drops Patchouli,
2 drops Rose Absolute,
6 drops Sweet Orange

To smooth wrinkles from dry skin:
2 drops Patchouli,
2 drops Jasmine Absolute, 6 drops Palmarosa

Himalayan Cedarwood (*Cedrus deodara*)

Majestically tall (reaching heights of up to 30m/100 ft), with strong branches that sweep to the ground, this aromatic tree dominates the skyline in countries such as India, Nepal and Tibet. Its inner wood is reddish-coloured and rich in essential oil, which has a soft, deep aroma and turns sharp and slightly sweet as it evaporates. In traditional Tibetan medicine, the wood and essential oil are used to help to treat respiratory issues, such as bronchitis, and urinary complaints, such as cystitis, as well as to heal damaged skin. The scent calms the breath and brings about a meditative state.

Safety first

Himalayan Cedarwood is non-toxic, non-irritant and non-sensitizing, so is safe for all skin types.

Supporting the spirit

- Used in a vaporizer, this essential oil helps to create a calm, peaceful mood, preparing you for meditation or yoga practice.
- This oil expands the breath and encourages a deep sense of inner peace and tranquillity.

Plant features: Tall, evergreen tree; aromatic wood

Part of plant used:
Needles

Oil produced in:
India, Nepal, Tibet

Extraction method:
Steam distillation

Special blends

Add these essential oils to 20ml/4 tsp carrier oil:

To relieve worry:
4 drops Himalayan Cedarwood, 4 drops Australian Sandalwood, 2 drops Patchouli

To calm chesty coughs:
4 drops Himalayan Cedarwood, 2 drops Myrrh, 4 drops Frankincense

Easing the mind

- To calm nerves, bathe with 2 drops Himalayan Cedarwood and 3 drops Lavender.
- To ease frustration caused by mental stress, vaporize 3 drops Himalayan Cedarwood and 3 drops Orange Leaf.
- To renew inner strength, mix Himalayan Cedarwood with Australian Sandalwood and Patchouli in a carrier oil (see first blend, left) and apply it whenever you feel anxious.

Healing the body

- To ease coughs, bronchitis and asthma, mix Himalayan Cedarwood with Myrrh and Frankincense in a carrier (see second blend, left) and rub it into the chest twice daily.
- To fight viruses, bathe with 2 drops Himalayan Cedarwood and 2 drops Black Pepper.
- To relieve a blocked nose or ease difficult breathing, try an inhalation with 3 drops Himalayan Cedarwood and 3 drops Lemon.

Keywords

Expansive

Grounding

Supportive

149

Myrrh *(Commiphora myrrha)*

Native to the deserts of Oman, Yemen, Ethiopia and Somalia, the tough myrrh shrub oozes a sticky reddish-orange gum. This gum seals the inner wood of the shrub, preventing moisture loss. In Western herbal medicine, myrrh gum is used to treat mouth ulcers, bleeding gums, skin wounds and chest infections. The oil has an unusually sharp, woody yet bittersweet aroma.

Plant features: Tough aromatic shrub with sharp needles

Part of plant used: Gum

Oil produced in: Somalia, Oman, Yemen, Ethiopia

Extraction method: Steam distillation

Safety first
• Myrrh oil is non-toxic, non-irritant and non-sensitizing, so is safe for all skin types.
• Do not use Myrrh oil during pregnancy.

Supporting the spirit
• This oil calms the breath, enhancing meditation.
• Myrrh creates a sense of inner peace and tranquillity.

Easing the mind
• To dissolve feelings of anger or hurt, bathe with 2 drops Myrrh and 4 drops Rose Geranium.

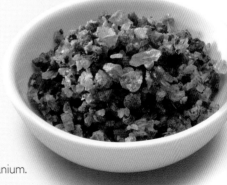

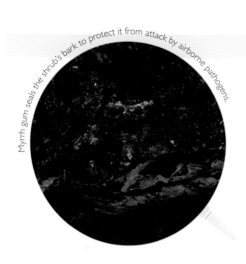

Myrrh gum seals the shrub's bark to protect it from attack by airborne pathogens.

Keywords

Soothing

Releasing

Opening

• To ease mental stress, vaporize 2 drops Myrrh and 4 drops Clove Bud.

Healing the body

• To soothe tight, chesty coughs, inhale 2 drops Myrrh and 4 drops Himalayan Cedarwood.
• To ease chest infections, mix Myrrh with Black Spruce and Laurel Leaf in a carrier (see first blend, right) and massage it into the chest.
• To repair a skin wound that is slow to heal, mix Myrrh with German Chamomile and Frankincense in a carrier (see second blend, right) and apply it to the wound twice daily.
• To draw out an infection, use a hot compress with 2 drops Myrrh and 2 drops Bergamot.

Special blends

Add these essential oils to 20ml/4 tsp carrier oil:

To soothe bronchitis or chest infections:
4 drops Myrrh, 2 drops Black Spruce, 4 drops Laurel Leaf

To heal skin wounds:
4 drops Myrrh, 2 drops German Chamomile, 4 drops Frankincense

Lemon-scented Eucalyptus (Eucalyptus citriodora)

One of 600 species of eucalyptus, the lemon-scented variety was originally native to Australia but is now cultivated in countries such as China, Brazil and Indonesia, too. This species is unusual among eucalyptus trees because, rather than having leaves with a penetrating, medicinal aroma, its leaves have a strong, lemony smell. This scent comes from a biochemical ingredient called citronellal, which is a highly effective mosquito repellent. The essential oil, from the leaves, has a gentle aroma that is soft and sweet, with fresh, citrusy notes.

Safety first

Lemon-scented Eucalyptus oil is non-toxic, non-irritant and non-sensitizing, so is safe for all skin types.

Supporting the spirit

- This essential oil will promote your awareness of your "inner child", as well as enhancing feelings of safety and trust in others.
- This oil encourages lightness of heart and spontaneous expressions of joy.

Plant features: Small tree with pinkish bark and pale green leaves

Part of plant used: Leaves

Oil produced in: Australia, China, Brazil, Indonesia

Extraction method: Steam distillation

Special blends

Add these essential oils to 20ml/4 tsp carrier oil:

To relieve coughs or colds in small children:
2 drops Lemon-scented Eucalyptus, 2 drops Lavender

To relieve the symptoms of asthma:
4 drops Lemon-scented Eucalyptus, 2 drops Benzoin Resinoid, 4 drops Myrrh

Easing the mind

- To lift depression, vaporize 3 drops Lemon-scented Eucalyptus and 4 drops Tangerine.
- To bring new hope and restore positive energy, bathe with 2 drops Lemon-scented Eucalyptus and 4 drops Sweet Orange.

Healing the body

- To ease chesty coughs, colds and sore throats in children aged between two and ten, mix Lemon-scented Eucalyptus with Lavender in a carrier oil (see first blend, left) and rub it into the chest, morning and night.
- To soothe the symptoms of asthma, mix Lemon-scented Eucalyptus in a carrier with Benzoin Resinoid and Myrrh (see second blend, left) and massage it into the chest twice a day.
- To clear up dandruff or soothe an irritated scalp, wash your hair with 2 drops Lemon-scented Eucalyptus in 5ml/1 tsp unscented shampoo daily.

Keywords
Soft
Gentle
Light

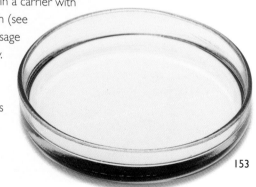

153

Eucalyptus (*Eucalyptus globulus*)

Also known as the "blue gum" or "Tasmanian Blue", this is the most common eucalyptus species in the world. The tree was originally native to Australia and is now naturalized in many countries, including Spain, China and Portugal. Its leaves are extremely rich in eucalyptol, used in cough medicines, as well as muscle-warming ointments and liniments. The essential oil itself contains about 70-per-cent eucalyptol, too, making it an effective remedy for chesty coughs. The oil has a clean, medicinal and penetrating aroma, with lovely fresh notes.

Safety first

- Used on the skin, this oil is non-toxic, non-irritant and non-sensitizing, so is safe for all skin types.
- No essential oil should be taken internally, but Eucalyptus can be particularly toxic. Always keep it away from small children.

Supporting the spirit

- Eucalyptus oil dissolves feelings of melancholy.
- This oil restores positive energy.

Plant features: Very tall tree with blue-green leaves

Part of plant used: Leaves

Oil produced in: Australia, Spain, China, Portugal

Extraction method: Steam distillation

Special blends

Add these essential oils to 20ml/4 tsp carrier oil:

To soothe dry or chesty coughs:
4 drops Eucalyptus, 2 drops Myrrh, 4 drops Himalayan Cedarwood

To warm and soothe painful muscles:
4 drops Eucalyptus, 2 drops Ginger, 4 drops Rosemary

Easing the mind

- To lift depression and bring a sense of release, vaporize 3 drops Eucalyptus and 3 drops Peppermint.
- To clear cluttered thoughts, take a bath with 2 drops Eucalyptus and 4 drops Frankincense.

Healing the body

- To ease breathing during colds, bronchitis, or episodes of sinusitis or hay fever, or to help to prevent airborne infection, vaporize 3 drops Eucalyptus and 3 drops Tea Tree.
- To ease coughs, mix Eucalyptus with Myrrh and Himalayan Cedarwood in a carrier oil (see first blend, left) and rub it into the chest, morning and evening.
- To clear blocked nasal passages, try an inhalation with 3 drops Eucalyptus and 3 drops Lavandin.
- To ease stiff or pulled muscles, mix Eucalyptus with Ginger and Rosemary in a carrier oil (see second blend, left) and rub it into the affected areas twice a day.

| **Keywords** |
| Clean |
| Fresh |
| Expansive |

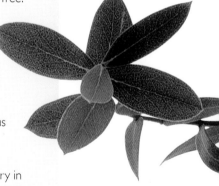

155

Laurel Leaf (*Laurus nobilis*)

The laurel tree grows all around the Mediterranean region, particularly in Spain, Greece, Morocco and parts of Eastern Europe, such as Hungary. This is the tree that gives us the "bay leaf", which is often used in cooking, and should not be confused with West Indian Bay (see pp.172–3). Laurel leaves are highly aromatic, and the essential oil obtained from them is beautiful, with a pungent young and fresh aroma and definite spicy undertones, growing sweeter as it evaporates.

Safety first

- This oil is non-toxic.
- Laurel Leaf is a potential irritant or sensitizer: avoid it in baths or massage if you have sensitive or allergy-prone skin.
- Do not use Laurel Leaf during pregnancy.

Supporting the spirit

- Laurel Leaf promotes the fire of creativity and renews inspiration.
- This oil transforms lethargy and low spirits, restoring enthusiasm for everything you do.

Plant features: Evergreen tree with dark green leaves

Part of plant used: Leaves

Oil produced in: Spain, Greece, Morocco, Hungary

Extraction method: Steam distillation

Special blends

Add these essential oils to 20ml/4 tsp carrier oil:

To boost self-confidence and help you to face adversity:
2 drops Laurel Leaf, 4 drops Myrtle, 4 drops Frankincense

To help the body to fight off flu:
2 drops Laurel Leaf, 4 drops Black Pepper, 4 drops Bergamot

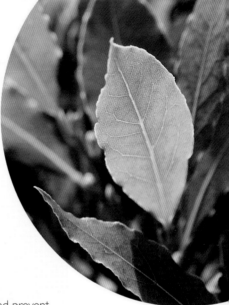

Easing the mind

- To build self-confidence and the strength to meet challenges, mix Laurel Leaf with Myrtle and Frankincense in a carrier oil (see first blend, left) for a daytime massage.
- To relieve feelings of hopelessness, vaporize 3 drops Laurel Leaf and 3 drops Bergamot.

Healing the body

- To build up the immune system and prevent the onset of viruses, such as colds and flu, take a daily bath with 3 drops Laurel Leaf and 3 drops Manuka.
- To fortify the body during flu, boosting the immune and respiratory systems, mix Laurel Leaf with Black Pepper and Bergamot in a carrier oil (see second blend, left) and rub it into the chest, morning and night.
- To clear sinusitis, try an inhalation of 2 drops Laurel Leaf and 4 drops Lemon.

Keywords

Bracing

Strengthening

Invigorating

157

Cajeput *(Melaleuca cajeputi)*

A vigorous tree with whitish, papery bark that peels away in strips, Cajeput is a member of the same botanical family as the tea tree (see pp.138–9) and niaouli (see pp.160–61). It is native to parts of Indonesia and Malaysia, as well as to Australia, where the leaves are regarded as a cure for colds, flu, bronchitis, headaches, and muscular and rheumatic problems. Because of its distant origins, Cajeput essential oil has been known in European herbal medicine only since the 17th century. It has a very pungent, penetrating, medicinal aroma, with lighter fruity notes.

Safety first

Cajeput is non-toxic and non-sensitizing, but it is mildly irritant, so avoid it in baths or massage if you have delicate or damaged skin.

Supporting the spirit

• Cajeput helps you to overcome a lack of energy and renews zest for life.

• This oil restores a sense of inner purpose during times when you feel lost or alone.

Plant features: Evergreen tree with pointed leaves

Part of plant used: Leaves

Oil produced in: Indonesia, Malaysia, Australia

Extraction method: Steam distillation

Special blends

Add these essential oils to 20ml/4 tsp carrier oil:

To boost the immune and respiratory systems during illness:
2 drops Cajeput,
4 drops Bergamot,
4 drops Laurel Leaf

To soothe muscle pain and backache:
2 drops Cajeput,
4 drops Nutmeg,
4 drops Cardamom

Easing the mind

- To clear mental muddle, vaporize 2 drops Cajeput and 4 drops Peppermint.
- To help to alleviate restlessness as a result of mental overload, take a bath with 1 drop Cajeput and 4 drops Australian Sandalwood.

Healing the body

- To clear blocked nasal passages, try an inhalation with 2 drops Cajeput and 4 drops Eucalyptus.
- To support the body's systems during colds or flu, bathe with 1 drop Cajeput and 4 drops Lavender; and/or mix Cajeput with Bergamot and Laurel Leaf in a carrier (see first blend, left) and rub the blend into your chest, morning and evening.
- To ease aching muscles, or to relieve backache, mix Cajeput with Nutmeg and Cardamom in a carrier oil (see second blend, left) and apply it with firm, soothing strokes, two or three times a day.

Keywords

Pungent

Warming

Strengthening

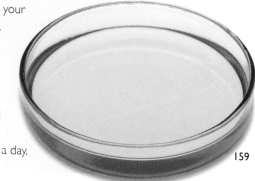

159

Niaouli (*Melaleuca quinquenervia*)

Naturally thriving in the swampy terrain of New South Wales and Queensland in Australia, this evergreen tree has been successfully introduced to Madagascar, a country that is now an important source of the essential oil. Niaouli oil is concentrated in the tree's bright green leaves and is extensively used in the pharmaceutical industry to make cough medicines, mouth sprays and gargles. In France, where medical doctors prescribe essential oils as natural antimicrobial remedies, Niaouli is an extremely popular choice for its antibacterial properties. It has a fresh, clearing and medicinal aroma, with sweeter notes as it evaporates.

Safety first

This essential oil is non-toxic, non-irritant and non-sensitizing, so is safe for all skin types.

Supporting the spirit

- Niaouli brings on feelings of expansion, giving you a sense of having "room to breathe".
- This oil helps to lighten emotional burdens and release tension.

Plant features: Evergreen tree with pointed leaves

Part of plant used: Leaves and twigs

Oil produced in: Australia, Madagascar

Extraction method: Steam distillation

Special blends

Add these essential oils to 20ml/4 tsp carrier oil:

To relieve hacking coughs and tightness in the chest:
2 drops Niaouli, 4 drops Myrrh, 4 drops Himalayan Cedarwood

To soothe the pain of aching muscles:
2 drops Niaouli, 4 drops Rosemary, 4 drops Spike Lavender

Easing the mind

- To ease frustration and clear the mind, vaporize 3 drops Niaouli and 3 drops Lemon.
- To relieve claustrophobia and panic attacks, place 2 drops Niaouli on a tissue and inhale.

Healing the body

- To relieve symptoms of acute bronchitis or sinusitis, try an inhalation with 3 drops Niaouli and 3 drops Eucalyptus.
- To soothe chesty or tight coughs, mix Niaouli with Myrrh and Himalayan Cedarwood in a carrier oil (see first blend, left) and rub it into the chest, morning and night.
- To draw out poison from insect bites, boils or skin infections, use a hot compress with 3 drops Niaouli and 3 drops Tea Tree.
- To relieve aching muscles, mix Niaouli, Rosemary and Spike Lavender in a carrier oil (see second blend, left) and rub the blend gently into the affected areas as necessary.

Keywords

Cleansing

Gentle

Uplifting

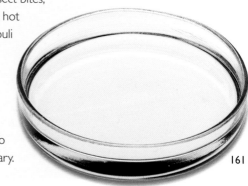

Myrtle (Myrtus communis)

The Ancient Greeks burned branches of this aromatic shrub as offerings to the goddess Artemis, who watched over the natural world. Today, in southern parts of France and Spain, the leaves are used to make a herbal infusion that helps women to balance their hormone cycles. The leaves also give us the essential oil, which has a fresh yet fruity aroma.

Plant features: Vigorous evergreen shrub

Part of plant used: Leaves

Oil produced in: Corsica, Spain

Extraction method: Steam distillation

Safety first
This oil is non-toxic, non-irritating and non-sensitizing, so is safe for all skin types.

Supporting the spirit
• Myrtle oil reconnects us with Nature.
• This oil encourages positive energy in personal relationships.

Easing the mind
• To improve mental focus, vaporize 3 drops Myrtle and 3 drops Rosemary.
• For support during life's transitions, bathe with 2 drops Myrtle and 2 drops Sweet Orange.

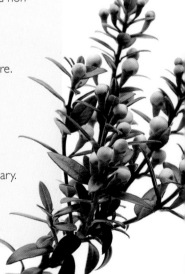

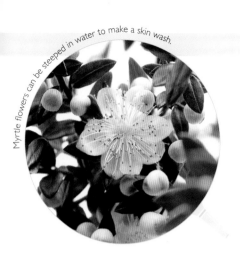

Myrtle flowers can be steeped in water to make a skin wash.

Keywords

Fresh

Light

Expansive

Healing the body

- To ease chesty coughs, try an inhalation with 3 drops Myrtle and 3 drops Laurel Leaf.
- To support the body during viral infections, such as flu, take a daily bath with 2 drops Myrtle and 2 drops Black Spruce.
- To overcome post-viral fatigue, mix Myrtle with Bergamot and Australian Sandalwood in a carrier oil (see first blend, right) and apply it gently to the skin using soothing strokes.
- To even out oily, combination or problem skin, mix Myrtle with Geranium and Mandarin, either in a carrier oil (see second blend, right) or in 20g/4 tsp Skin Mousse (see pp.42–3), and apply it to your face, morning and night.

Special blends

Add these essential oils to 20ml/4 tsp carrier oil:

To raise low energy:
4 drops Myrtle, 2 drops Bergamot, 4 drops Australian Sandalwood

To balance oily, combination or problem skin:
4 drops Myrtle, 2 drops Geranium, 4 drops Mandarin

Black Spruce (*Picea mariana*)

Native to Canada and the northern US, the black spruce tree has been valued for hundreds of years as a remedy for respiratory complaints, flu and rheumatic conditions. Native Americans also smeared the tree's resin onto their skin to keep stinging insects at bay. The essential oil comes from the highly aromatic needles; it has a rich, fresh yet smoky aroma with a strong, sharp, resiny tinge.

Plant features: Tall evergreen spruce tree

Part of plant used: Needles

Oil produced in: Canada, US

Extraction method: Steam distillation

Safety first

- Black Spruce oil is non-toxic, non-irritating and non-sensitizing, so is safe for all skin types.
- There is some evidence of sensitization to Black Spruce when using older bottles of the oil. If you store your oil at or above 10°C/55°F, keep it no longer than six months. In the refrigerator, it will last for a year.

Supporting the spirit

- Black Spruce essential oil helps to deepen the connection with your "inner self".
- This oil grounds and stabilizes the body's energy field or aura, making you feel balanced.

Special blends

Add these essential oils to 20ml/4 tsp carrier oil:

To dispel the physical effects of mental stress:
2 drops Black Spruce,
4 drops Spanish Sage,
4 drops Sweet Orange

To ease stubborn, phlegmy coughs:
4 drops Black Spruce,
2 drops Laurel Leaf,
4 drops Frankincense

Easing the mind

- To soothe persistent stress, take a bath with 2 drops Black Spruce and 4 drops Lavender.
- To ease mental stress characterized by physical tension, mix Black Spruce with Spanish Sage and Sweet Orange in a carrier oil (see first blend, left) and rub it into your shoulders, or wherever feels good.

Healing the body

- To soothe asthma, vaporize 3 drops Black Spruce and 3 drops Himalayan Cedarwood.
- To loosen mucusy coughs, mix Black Spruce with Laurel Leaf and Frankincense in a carrier oil (see second blend, left) and rub it into the chest, morning and night.
- To ease the body during colds or flu, take a bath with 2 drops Black Spruce and 4 drops Manuka.
- To ease muscular aches and pains, bathe with 2 drops Black Spruce and 2 drops Vetiver.

Keywords

Fresh

Bracing

Strengthening

Benzoin Resinoid *(Styrax benzoin)*

Found in various parts of tropical Asia, such as Java and Sumatra, the benzoin tree produces a sticky, reddish-brown resin, which is extremely aromatic, with strong vanilla and spice notes. In the West, this resin is best known as the main ingredient in "Friar's Balsam", a traditional remedy for respiratory problems. The resin is soaked in chemical solvents to produce a thick, reddish liquid called Benzoin Resinoid, which is not actually an essential oil, but an aromatic extract. When added to a vegetable carrier oil, such as Sweet Almond, Benzoin Resinoid turns the blend slightly cloudy.

Plant features: Tall tropical tree with pale green leaves

Part of plant used: Resin

Oil produced in: Tropical Asia

Extraction method: Solvent processing

Safety first
Benzoin Resinoid is non-toxic and non-irritant, but it is a mild sensitizer: avoid it if you have sensitive or allergy-prone skin.

Supporting the spirit
• Benzoin Resinoid warms and strengthens the heart and opens it to receive love.

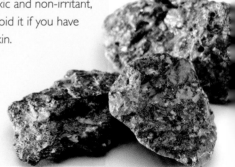

• Benzoin Resinoid creates a profound feeling of inner sweetness and tranquillity.

Easing the mind
• To calm and soothe deep emotional stress, vaporize 3 drops Benzoin Resinoid and 3 drops Cardamom.
• To relieve feelings of sadness, mix Benzoin Resinoid with May Chang and Neroli in a carrier oil (see first blend, right) and use gentle strokes to ease it into your body.

Healing the body
• To ease spasmodic coughs, bronchitis or asthma, mix Benzoin Resinoid with Myrtle and Myrrh in a carrier oil (see second blend, right) and apply it your chest, twice daily.
• To soothe a sore throat or laryngitis, try an inhalation with 2 drops Benzoin Resinoid and 4 drops Australian Sandalwood.
• To heal cracked or damaged skin, or eczema, apply 2 drops Benzoin Resinoid, 2 drops German Chamomile and 6 drops Lavender in 20g/4 tsp Skin Mousse (see pp.42–3).

Keywords

Warming

Sweet

Supportive

Special blends

Add the following to 20ml/4 tsp carrier oil:

To lift the spirits and relieve vulnerability:
2 drops Benzoin Resinoid, 4 drops May Chang, 4 drops Neroli

To relieve hacking coughs:
2 drops Benzoin Resinoid, 4 drops Myrtle, 4 drops Myrrh

167

Thyme *(Thymus vulgaris* – Linalool chemotype)

This popular herb has small, highly aromatic leaves, and spikes of tiny pink flowers in high summer. Originally native to the Mediterranean, it is now grown in many hot, dry climates. Plants from different locations produce Thyme essential oils with varied chemical constituents; these oils are known as "chemotypes". One of the safest and most effective chemotypes is Thyme Linalool, from France. This mild oil is gentle on the skin, with a soft, herbal and pungent fragrance. From good suppliers, the name Thyme Linalool will appear on the bottle's label. Avoid Red Thyme essential oil – it contains thymol, which irritates the skin. Thyme Linalool is profiled below.

Plant features:
Low-growing herb

Part of plant used:
Leaves

Oil produced in:
France

Extraction method:
Steam distillation

Safety first
This oil is non-toxic, non-irritating and non-sensitizing so is safe for all skin types.

Supporting the spirit
• Thyme creates a feeling of release and calm.

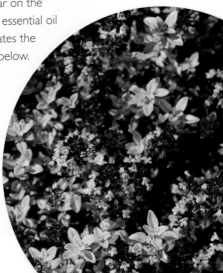

168

• This oil helps to dissolve feelings of heaviness and restriction.

Easing the mind
• To lift depression, vaporize 3 drops Thyme and 3 drops Sweet Orange.
• To help to ground and focus mental awareness, take a bath with 2 drops Thyme and 4 drops Bergamot Mint.

Healing the body
• To unblock the respiratory passages during colds and flu, try an inhalation with 3 drops Thyme and 3 drops Peppermint.
• To support the body's systems during viral infections, such as colds and flu, mix Thyme with Lemon and Clove Bud in a carrier oil (see first blend, right) and rub it into the chest and neck, morning and night.
• To overcome post-viral fatigue and low energy, mix Thyme with Mandarin and Cardamom in a carrier oil (see second blend, right) and massage it into your body whenever you need a boost.

Keywords

Soothing

Warming

Gentle

Special blends

Add these essential oils to 20ml/4 tsp carrier oil:

To boost immunity and support the body during viruses:
4 drops Thyme,
4 drops Lemon,
2 drops Clove Bud

To relieve post-viral fatigue and raise energy:
4 drops Thyme,
4 drops Mandarin,
2 drops Cardamom

169

Cinnamon Leaf (*Cinnamonum verum*)

Native to Sri Lanka, Madagascar, southern India and other parts of southeast Asia, cinnamon trees are famous for their spice, which as well as being a flavouring, has had medicinal uses for centuries to help circulatory, digestive and immune-deficiency problems. It comes from the aromatic, dried inner bark of the tree, which can also yield an essential oil. However, this oil is far too irritant to use in aromatherapy. Fortunately, the leaves of the tree are also aromatic, and yield a much milder essential oil with a soft, spicy and warm fragrance.

Safety first
- Cinnamon Leaf oil is non-toxic.
- This oil can be a mild irritant or sensitizer: avoid it in baths or massage if you have sensitive or allergy-prone skin.

Supporting the spirit
- Cinnamon Leaf transforms low vitality and lack of motivation into a zest for life.
- This essential oil boosts creativity and stimulates new ideas.

Plant features: Bushy, aromatic, evergreen tree

Part of plant used: Leaves

Oil produced in: Sri Lanka, Madagascar, Southeast Asia

Extraction method: Steam distillation

Special blends

Add these essential oils to 20ml/4 tsp carrier oil:

To boost blood-flow to the extremities:
2 drops Cinnamon Leaf, 4 drops Ginger, 4 drops Lavandin

To relieve indigestion:
2 drops Cinnamon Leaf, 4 drops Coriander Seed, 4 drops Tangerine

Easing the mind

- To lift depression and
  ease away any sense of
  hopelessness, vaporize
  2 drops Cinnamon Leaf and
  4 drops Sweet Orange.
- To relieve mental exhaustion
  and enable fresh thinking, place
  1 drop Cinnamon Leaf on a tissue
  and inhale.

Healing the body

- To stimulate the circulation and warm cold
  legs and feet, mix Cinnamon Leaf with Ginger
  and Lavandin in a carrier oil (see first blend,
  left) and rub it into legs and feet twice a day.
- To support the body through viral infections,
  such as flu, take a daily bath with 1 drop
  Cinnamon Leaf and 3 drops Ginger.
- To ease indigestion caused by physical stress,
  mix Cinnamon Leaf with Coriander Seed
  and Tangerine in a carrier oil (see second
  blend, left) and apply it to the abdomen using
  clockwise strokes.

Keywords

Fiery

Energizing

Strengthening

West Indian Bay (*Pimenta racemosa*)

Not to be confused with laurel (see pp.156–7), this aromatic tree has large, tough leaves and fragrant berries. Since the 18th century, the fragrance of West Indian Bay has enhanced many cosmetic products and pungent aftershaves for men. The tree's leaves yield the essential oil, which contains powerful constituents – so you need use very little in aromatherapy for therapeutic effect. Its vibrant scent, which is spicy and fresh, with rich, resiny notes as it evaporates, will appeal to you if you don't like lighter, sweeter essential oils.

Safety first
- West Indian Bay oil is non-toxic and non-sensitizing.
- This oil may be irritating to the mucous membranes (see p.276): avoid it in baths or inhalations.

Supporting the spirit
- West Indian Bay inspires courage and generates the energy to take action.
- This oil instantly invigorates the spirit.

Plant features: Evergreen tree with large leaves

Part of plant used: Leaves

Oil produced in: West Indies

Extraction method: Steam distillation

Special blends

Add these essential oils to 20ml/4 tsp carrier oil:

To ease depression or lack of self-worth:
2 drops West Indian Bay,
4 drops Sweet Orange,
4 drops Neroli

To boost circulation and warm the limbs:
2 drops West Indian Bay,
4 drops Cubeb Pepper,
4 drops Bergamot

Easing the mind

- To transform apathy and listlessness into renewed zest for life, vaporize 2 drops West Indian Bay and 2 drops Cinnamon Leaf.
- To relieve depression and overcome a lack of self-worth, mix West Indian Bay with Sweet Orange and Neroli in a carrier oil (see first blend, left) and smooth the blend gently into your body, whenever you feel the need.

Healing the body

- To boost the circulation and warm cold limbs or stiff, aching muscles, mix West Indian Bay with Cubeb Pepper and Bergamot in a carrier (see second blend, left) and rub the blend into the affected areas twice a day.
- To support the body's systems during flu, vaporize 2 drops West Indian bay and 4 drops Kanuka.
- To treat dandruff, add 2 drops West Indian Bay to 1 tsp/5ml plain shampoo; rub into the scalp, and rinse, daily.

Keywords
Bracing
Pungent
Powerful

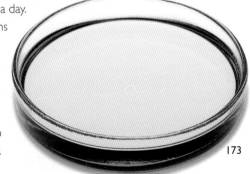

173

Cubeb Seed (*Piper cubeba*)

Cubeb is a climbing vine from Indonesia that produces stems up to 7m/20ft tall, with long, heart-shaped leaves. A close relative of black pepper (see pp.176–7), cubeb is unusual because its orange-brown peppercorns retain their stems, giving the spice its common name of "tailed pepper". In traditional Indonesian medicine, the dried peppercorns are used to ease urinary complaints, such as cystitis, as well as respiratory and circulatory problems. Cubeb Seed essential oil has a soft fragrance, with a citrusy tang and soft, spicy hints as it evaporates. Unlike other fiery spices, it has a gently nurturing effect.

Safety first

This oil is non-toxic, non-irritating and non-sensitizing, so is safe for all skin types.

Supporting the spirit

• Cubeb Seed essential oil softly envelops and nurtures the heart.
• This oil will help you to express joy and show spontaneity.

Plant features: Tall, vigorous climbing vine

Part of plant used: Dried fruit

Oil produced in: Indonesia

Extraction method: Steam distillation

Special blends

Add these essential oils to 20ml/4 tsp carrier oil.

To boost self-belief and improve libido:
4 drops Cubeb Seed, 2 drops Jasmine Absolute, 4 drops Australian Sandalwood

To warm the circulation and ease muscle pain:
4 drops Cubeb Seed, 2 drops Ginger, 4 drops Cardamom

Easing the mind

- To revitalize low mental energy, bathe with 4 drops Cubeb Seed and 2 drops Cardamom.
- To help to restore self-confidence and improve sexual energy, mix Cubeb Seed with Jasmine Absolute and Australian Sandalwood in a carrier (see first blend, left) and smooth it into your body – during the evening is best.

Healing the body

- To boost the circulation and ease aching muscles, mix Cubeb Seed, Ginger and Cardamom in a carrier oil (see second blend, left) and apply it twice a day.
- To support the body during flu, take a bath with 4 drops Cubeb Seed and 2 drops Bergamot.
- To ease bronchitis and chesty coughs, inhale 2 drops Cubeb Seed and 4 drops Himalayan Cedarwood.

Keywords

Gentle

Fortifying

Supportive

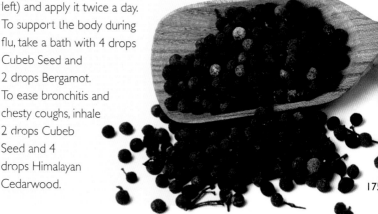

175

Black Pepper (*Piper nigrum*)

Native to both India and Indonesia, fiery black pepper has been used therapeutically for more than 4,000 years. In traditional Ayurvedic medicine, black pepper was thought not only to warm the body, but also to re-energize the system and restore vitality. Peppercorns are the ripe fruit of the pepper vine, turning black as they dry in the sun. They contain Black Pepper essential oil, which has a spicy, pungent aroma, with lingering warm, woody notes.

Plant features:
Vigorous climbing vine

Part of plant used:
Dried fruit

Oil produced in:
India, Indonesia

Extraction method:
Steam distillation

Safety first
- Black Pepper oil is non-toxic.
- This oil can be mildly irritant or sensitizing: avoid it in baths or massage if you have sensitive or allergy-prone skin.

Supporting the spirit
- Black Pepper dissolves spiritual exhaustion, breaking through self-doubt.
- This oil revives inner conviction and gives the strength to act.

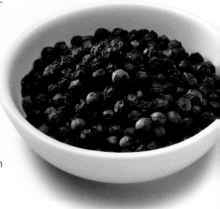

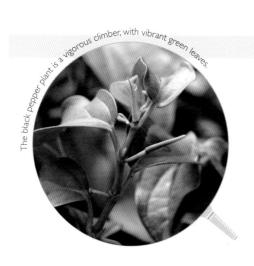

The black pepper plant is a vigorous climber, with vibrant green leaves.

Keywords

Fiery

Summery

Stimulating

Easing the mind

- To cope with ongoing mental stress, vaporize 3 drops Black Pepper and 3 drops Mandarin.
- To restore sexual energy and warm the emotions, take a bath with 2 drops Black Pepper and 2 drops Rose Absolute.

Healing the body

- To ease stiff muscles, apply Black Pepper, West Indian Bay and Spike Lavender mixed in a carrier oil (see first blend, right) twice a day.
- To improve sluggish digestion, mix Black Pepper with Ginger and Bergamot Mint in a carrier oil (see second blend, right) and apply, using clockwise abdominal massage.

Special blends

Add these essential oils to 20ml/4 tsp carrier oil:

To ease muscle pain:
2 drops Black Pepper,
2 drops West Indian Bay,
6 drops Spike Lavender

To stimulate digestion and ease constipation:
2 drops Black Pepper,
4 drops Ginger, 4 drops
Bergamot Mint

177

Clove Bud (*Syzygium aromaticum*)

The clove tree is an intensely aromatic, evergreen tree from Indonesia, producing the clove "nails" that are so well-known as a spice. For centuries, dried cloves have been chewed to release their essential oil, which has a strong numbing effect on toothache and is still used as an antiseptic pain-relieving remedy in dentistry. The essential oil from ripe cloves is too strong to use in aromatherapy, but the unripe buds of the flowers produce an oil that is gentler, yet still wonderfully fresh, warming and spicy.

Safety first

- Clove Bud oil is non-toxic.
- This essential oil can be mildly irritant or sensitizing: avoid using it in baths or for massage if you have sensitive or allergy-prone skin.

Supporting the spirit

- Clove Bud essential oil expands and enhances inner strength and vision.
- This oil encourages inspired action and the pursuit of your true path.

Plant features: Evergreen tree with rich green leaves and pink flowers

Part of plant used: Buds

Oil produced in: Indonesia

Extraction method: Steam distillation

Special blends

Add these essential oils to 20ml/4 tsp carrier oil:

To improve blood-flow to aching muscles:
2 drops Clove Bud,
2 drops Cinnamon Leaf,
6 drops Mandarin

To boost the immune system:
2 drops Clove Bud,
4 drops Cardamom,
4 drops Bergamot

Easing the mind

- To strengthen mental weakness and relieve feelings of inadequacy, vaporize 3 drops Clove Bud and 3 drops Tangerine.
- To improve concentration and focus, place 2 drops Clove Bud on a tissue, and inhale.

Healing the body

- To stimulate the circulation and relieve muscular pains and osteoarthritis, mix Clove Bud with Cinnamon Leaf and Mandarin in a carrier oil (see first blend, left) and rub into the affected areas two or three times a day.
- To support immunity during chronic viral infections, such as glandular fever, gently massage in Clove Bud with Cardamom and Bergamot in a carrier oil (see second blend, left).
- To ease chesty coughs and open the airways, try an inhalation with 2 drops Clove Bud and 4 drops Myrtle.

Keywords
Dynamic
Fiery
Energizing

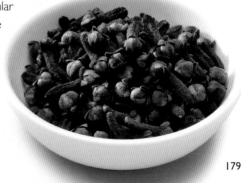

179

Linaloe Wood (*Bursera delpechiana* syn. *Bursera glabrifolia*)

Linaloe Wood essential oil is quite new to the aromatherapist's kit; practitioners use it as a sustainable alternative to the oil from the endangered Brazilian Rosewood tree (*Aniba rosaeodora*). Linaloe Wood oil resembles Rosewood quite closely in its chemical constituents, and has a similar sweet, woody and soft aroma. The linaloe tree has reddish branches and bushy foliage. When the wood is fresh, it has no odour, but when the trunks and branches are felled and left in the sun, the aroma develops. Older trunks yield up to 12 per cent of their weight in essential oil.

Safety first

Linaloe Wood essential oil is non-toxic, non-irritating and non-sensitizing, so is safe for all skin types.

Supporting the spirit

- Linaloe Wood oil brings a sense of inner peace and harmony.
- This essential oil helps to bring erratic energy back to a point of stillness.

Plant features: Tropical tree with vivid green leaves

Part of plant used: Dried wood

Oil produced in: Mexico

Extraction method: Steam distillation

Special blends

Add these essential oils to 20ml/4 tsp carrier oil:

To boost the immune system:
4 drops Linaloe Wood, 4 drops Cardamom, 2 drops Bergamot

To nurture the body through chronic fatigue or post-viral conditions:
4 drops Linaloe Wood, 2 drops Neroli, 4 drops Tangerine

Easing the mind
- To lift depression, vaporize 4 drops Linaloe Wood and 2 drops Frankincense.
- To relax the mind, take a bath with 4 drops Linaloe Wood and 2 drops Lavender.

Healing the body
- To fortify the immune system, thus preventing viral infections, such as colds and flu, mix Linaloe Wood with Cardamom and Bergamot in a carrier oil (see first blend, left) and massage the blend into your chest daily.
- To support recovery from chronic fatigue and post-viral conditions, mix Linaloe Wood, Neroli and Tangerine in a carrier oil (see second blend, left) and apply it to your skin using gentle strokes.
- To condition normal or dry skins, add 2 drops Linaloe Wood, 4 drops Geranium and 4 drops Australian Sandalwood to 20g/4 tsp Skin Mousse (see pp.42–3) and apply it nightly to your face.

Keywords

Soft

Supportive

Nurturing

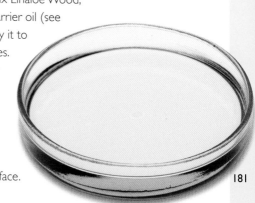

181

Lemon *(Citrus limon)*

Like all citrus species, lemon trees are evergreen, producing several crops of fruit in a year. In southern European countries, such as Spain and Italy, where lemon trees thrive, the fruit is regarded as a cure-all, especially for fevers and viral infections. The fruit's peel is full of tiny sacs that contain the essential oil. The aroma is intensely fruity, citrusy, zesty and fresh, with wonderful light, fizzy top notes.

Plant features: Evergreen tree with yellow fruit

Part of plant used: Fruit peel

Oil produced in: Spain, Italy

Extraction method: Expression

Safety first
• This oil is non-toxic and non-sensitizing.
• The oil can be a mild irritant: avoid it in baths or massage if you have sensitive skin.
• Lemon is phototoxic, so avoid using it on your skin if you are going out in the sun.

Supporting the spirit
• Lemon lifts dark moods, renewing zest for life.
• This oil restores focus, aiding problem-solving.

Easing the mind
• To clear a muddled head, vaporize 3 drops Lemon with 3 drops Eucalyptus.

Special blends

Add these essential oils to 20ml/4 tsp carrier oil.

To improve energy and relieve post-viral fatigue:
4 drops Lemon, 4 drops Myrtle, 2 drops Manuka

To relieve tiredness in late pregnancy (after 6 months):
2 drops Lemon, 2 drops Lavender

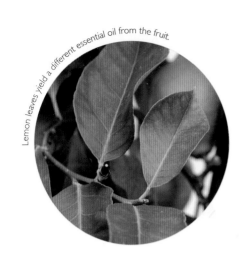

Lemon leaves yield a different essential oil from the fruit.

Keywords

Fresh

Cleansing

Bright

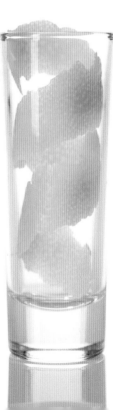

- To regulate mood swings, especially after the second trimester of pregnancy, bathe with 2 drops Lemon and 2 drops Geranium.

Healing the body

- To fight flu or a cold, try an inhalation of 3 drops Lemon and 3 drops Tea Tree.
- To overcome post-viral fatigue or raise low energy, mix Lemon with Myrtle and Manuka in a carrier oil (see first blend, left) and apply it to your skin whenever you need a boost.
- To relieve physical tiredness in late pregnancy, mix Lemon with Lavender in a carrier oil (see second blend, left), and ask a friend or partner to rub the blend gently into your lower back.

Immortelle *(Helichrysum italicum)*

A highly scented herb native to the southern Mediterranean, Immortelle also goes by the name "Everlasting". This is because the flowering tops keep their yellow colour, even as they dry out when the plant matures. Immortelle has a long tradition of therapeutic use, in particular to help chronic immune complaints, and headaches and skin problems. The oil is often reddish in colour and has a warm fragrance: rich and honey-sweet, with medicinal undertones and woody notes.

Plant features: Aromatic herb with greyish foliage

Part of plant used: Flowering tops

Oil produced in: Italy, Corsica

Extraction method: Steam distillation

Safety first
Immortelle oil is non-toxic, non-irritating and non-sensitizing, so is safe for all skin types.

Supporting the spirit
• Immortelle oil brings a feeling of deep peace and spiritual connection.
• This oil opens the heart to love and helps to heal emotional wounds.

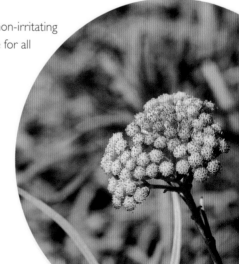

Easing the mind

- To diffuse anger or destructive feelings and restore inner calm, mix Immortelle with Rose Absolute and Australian Sandalwood in a carrier oil (see first blend, right) and rub the blend into your neck and shoulders.
- To soothe away deep emotional stress linked to the past, take a bath with 2 drops Immortelle and 2 drops Rose Absolute.

Healing the body

- To support the body through post-viral fatigue and convalescence, mix Immortelle with Ravensara and Lemon in a carrier oil (see second blend, right) and gently smooth it into your body as needed.
- To ease mucusy coughs, try an inhalation with 2 drops Immortelle and 4 drops Myrrh.
- To repair skin that has been damaged by psoriasis, eczema or ulceration, add 2 drops Immortelle, 4 drops Roman Chamomile and 4 drops Frankincense to 20g/4 tsp Skin Mousse (see pp.42–3) and apply it to the affected areas daily.

Keywords

Protective

Warming

Uplifting

Special blends

Add these essential oils to 20ml/4 tsp carrier oil:

To ease away anger and frustration:
2 drops Immortelle,
2 drops Rose Absolute,
6 drops Australian Sandalwood

To support the immune system through chronic viral illness:
2 drops Immortelle,
4 drops Ravensara,
4 drops Lemon

185

Kanuka *(Kunzea ericoides)*

Kanuka is a close relative of manuka (see pp.190–91). Both shrubs are native to New Zealand and valued by the Maoris for their medicinal effects, helping to boost immunity, and relieve sore joints and muscles. As yet, kanuka is not commercially cultivated, so the essential oil comes solely from fast-growing, tenacious wild plants. Practitioners with a more energy-based approach to aromatherapy believe that oil from self-propagating plants is more powerful than that from cultivated sources. Kanuka essential oil has a sweet, sharp aroma, with an unusual banana-like mid-note.

Safety first
- Kanuka oil is non-toxic and non-irritant.
- This oil can be a mild sensitizer: avoid it in baths or massage if you have sensitive skin.

Supporting the spirit
- Kanuka refreshes the human energy field or aura, bringing a sense of lightness.
- This essential oil encourages clear self-expression.

Plant features: Vigorous evergreen shrub

Part of plant used: Leaves and twigs

Oil produced in: New Zealand

Extraction method: Steam distillation

Special blends

Add these essential oils to 20ml/4 tsp carrier oil:

To ease persistent or ongoing mental stress:
2 drops Kanuka, 4 drops May Chang, 4 drops Linaloe Wood

To boost energy levels and alleviate post-viral fatigue:
2 drops Kanuka, 4 drops Cardamom, 4 drops Mandarin

Kanuka

Easing the mind

- To ease anxiety, vaporize
  2 drops Kanuka with
  4 drops Sweet Orange.
- To relieve chronic mental
  stress, mix Kanuka with May
  Chang and Linaloe Wood in a
  carrier oil (see first blend, left)
  and massage the blend gently
  into your neck and shoulders.

Healing the body

- To support the body's systems through
  viruses such as flu, take a daily bath with
  2 drops Kanuka, 2 drops Black Pepper
  and 2 drops Bergamot.
- To raise low energy levels and help to
  overcome post-viral fatigue, mix Kanuka
  with Cardamom and Mandarin in a carrier
  oil (see second blend, left) and massage it
  into your body as needed.
- To heal athlete's foot, soak your feet in
  2 drops Kanuka added to a small bowl
  of warm water.

Keywords

Fresh

Light

Clearing

Lemon Tea Tree (*Leptospermum petersonii*)

Native to Queensland and New South Wales in Australia, this lemon-scented variety of tea tree (see pp.138–9) has narrow, pointed dark-green leaves that contain the lemony antibacterial compounds citral and citronellal. In Australia, the tree is popular in gardens as hedging or screens – not only does it look attractive, but its lemon fragrance acts as an insect repellent. Lemon Tea Tree essential oil has a sweet, light and lemony aroma, with fresh, soft notes as it evaporates.

Safety first

- Lemon Tea Tree oil is non-toxic.
- This oil can be a mild irritant and sensitizer: avoid it in baths or massage if you have sensitive or allergy-prone skin.

Supporting the spirit

- Lemon Tea Tree spreads a feeling of positive energy and will give you a sense of being bathed in light.
- This oil lifts heavy moods and stimulates you to explore new directions.

Plant features: Evergreen tree with dark green leaves

Part of plant used: Leaves

Oil produced in: Australia

Extraction method: Steam distillation

Special blends

Add these essential oils to 20ml/4 tsp carrier oil:

To lift energy, especially after a viral illness:
2 drops Lemon Tea Tree,
4 drops Lavender,
4 drops Sweet Marjoram

To ease anxiety-related indigestion:
2 drops Lemon Tea Tree,
4 drops Coriander Seed,
4 drops Orange Leaf

Easing the mind

- To ease depression and raise low self-confidence, take a bath with 2 drops Lemon Tea Tree and 2 drops Neroli.
- To reduce mental overload, vaporize 3 drops Lemon Tea Tree and 3 drops Spearmint.

Healing the body

- To support the body through colds or flu, vaporize 3 drops Lemon Tea Tree and 3 drops Ravensara (this combination also makes an effective inhalation).
- To relieve post-viral symptoms and boost energy, mix Lemon Tea Tree with Lavender and Sweet Marjoram in a carrier oil (see first blend, left) and gently rub the blend into your skin whenever you need a lift.
- To soothe indigestion caused by emotional stress, mix Lemon Tea Tree with Coriander Seed and Orange Leaf in a carrier oil (see second blend, left) and rub it into your abdomen, using clockwise strokes, twice daily.

Keywords

Bright

Fresh

Light

Manuka (*Leptospermum scoparium*)

This evergreen shrub is vigorous and vibrant, with beautiful pink flowers. Native to New Zealand, manuka is a well-known source of honey that fortifies the immune system. The plant is not commercially cultivated. Instead, the essential oil comes from leaves and twigs that are collected from wild plants. The oil has an unusually rich, spicy and herbaceous fragrance.

Plant features: Evergreen shrub with pink flowers

Part of plant used: Leaves and twigs

Oil produced in: New Zealand

Extraction method: Steam distillation

Safety first
Manuka oil is non-toxic, non-irritating and non-sensitizing, so is safe for all skin types.

Supporting the spirit
• Manuka promotes inner strength and the courage to take action.
• This oil protects against negative external influences.

Easing the mind
• To soothe vulnerability, take a bath containing 2 drops Manuka and 4 drops Lavender.

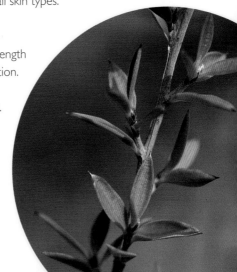

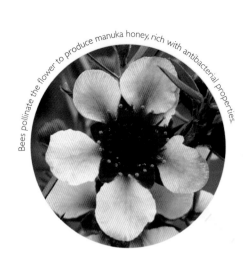

Bees pollinate the flower to produce manuka honey, rich with antibacterial properties.

Keywords

Protective

Strengthening

Warming

• To calm nervous tension, mix Manuka, Rose Geranium and Bergamot in a carrier (see first blend, right) and apply it gently to tense areas.

Healing the body

• To relieve cold symptoms, take a bath with 2 drops Manuka and 4 drops Cubeb Pepper.
• To restore energy after a virus, massage in a blend of Manuka, Clove Bud and Cardamom in a carrier oil (see second blend, right).
• To heal cuts and insect bites, apply 2 drops Manuka, 4 drops Myrrh and 4 drops Lavender in 20g/4 tsp Skin Mousse (see pp.42–3).
• To ease muscular stiffness, take a bath with 4 drops Manuka and 2 drops Vetiver.

Special blends

Add these essential oils to 20ml/4 tsp carrier oil:

To relieve extreme nervous tension:
2 drops Manuka, 4 drops Rose Geranium, 4 drops Bergamot

To restore physical energy following a viral illness:
4 drops Manuka, 2 drops Clove Bud, 4 drops Cardamom

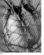

Black Cumin Seed (*Nigella sativa*)

Not to be confused with the well-known cumin seed curry spice (*Cuminum cyminium*), black cumin is a creeping plant with grey-green leaves. Its flowers become pods containing the aromatic seeds. The process of pressing these seeds yields an oil rich in omega-3 and -6 fatty acids; distilling them releases the essential oil. Recent Egyptian research has shown that Black Cumin Seed is one of the most potent natural antibacterial and antiviral essential oils. The fragrance is pungent, spicy and heavy – you need only 1 drop in baths, inhalations or blends.

Plant features: Low creeper with blue flowers

Part of plant used: Seeds

Oil produced in: Egypt

Extraction method: Steam distillation

Safety first
- This oil is non-toxic and non-irritant.
- This oil may be sensitizing: avoid it in baths or massage if you have sensitive skin.

Supporting the spirit
- Black Cumin Seed protects the spirit against negative external influences, such as others' bad-temperedness.

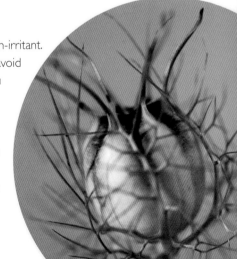

192

• This essential oil brings vitality to the "subtle body" – the home of your vital energy or life force – especially during illness.

Easing the mind

• To soothe mental weakness or exhaustion, mix Black Cumin Seed with Vetiver and Lavender in a carrier oil (see first blend, right) and rub it into your body each morning.

• To heal numbed emotions, vaporize 1 drop Black Cumin Seed and 4 drops Cardamom.

Healing the body

• To strengthen immunity during flu, try an inhalation with 1 drop Black Cumin seed, 2 drops Vetiver and 3 drops Cubeb Pepper.

• To assist recovery from chronic immune infections, such as glandular fever, as well as chronic fatigue, mix Black Cumin Seed, Lemon and Manuka in a carrier oil (see second blend, right) and apply it to the chest, neck and shoulders, morning and night.

• To combat urinary infections, bathe with 1 drop Black Cumin Seed and 3 drops Tea Tree.

Keywords

Powerful

Pungent

Protective

Special blends

Add these essential oils to 20ml/4 tsp carrier oil:

To ease mental exhaustion:
1 drop Black Cumin Seed, 2 drops Vetiver, 6 drops Lavender

To help overcome chronic illness:
1 drop Black Cumin Seed, 4 drops Lemon, 4 drops Manuka

Ravensara (*Ravensara aromatica*)

Native to Madagascar, ravensara is a member of the same tree family as may chang (see pp.214–15). Ravensara essential oil helps to boost the body's immune response and also assists with post-viral recovery. It has a soft, eucalyptus-like aroma, with fresh, herbal notes. When you buy this oil, make sure that the botanical name is *Ravensara aromatica* as another species, *Ravensara anisata*, is also available as an essential oil, but this oil contains ingredients that may damage the skin.

Safety first
Ravensara oil is non-toxic, non-irritating and non-sensitizing, so is safe for all skin types.

Supporting the spirit
• Ravensara oil restores self-confidence.
• This essential oil deepens inner focus in order to achieve spiritual and life goals.

Easing the mind
• To ease nervous exhaustion, take a bath with 4 drops Ravensara and 2 drops Vetiver.

Plant features: Tropical evergreen tree

Part of plant used: Leaves

Oil produced in: Madagascar

Extraction method: Steam distillation

Special blends

Add these essential oils to 20ml/4 tsp carrier oil:

To ease ongoing anxiety and exhaustion:
2 drops Ravensara,
2 drops Rose Absolute,
6 drops Tangerine

To help the body to recover from viral illness:
4 drops Ravensara,
4 drops Linaloe Wood,
2 drops Neroli

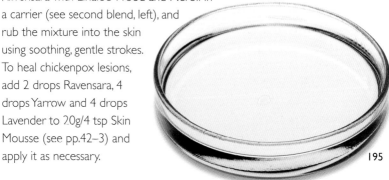

• To soothe emotional weakness and chronic stress, mix Ravensara with Rose Absolute and Tangerine in a carrier oil (see first blend, left) and, if possible, ask a friend to apply it in a soothing back massage, or otherwise apply it gently in self-massage.

Healing the body

• To help the body to fight flu, bathe with 2 drops Ravensara and 4 drops Cardamom.

• To ease tight or painful coughs, try an inhalation of 3 drops Ravensara and 3 drops Himalayan Cedarwood.

• To support post-viral convalescence, mix Ravensara with Linaloe Wood and Neroli in a carrier (see second blend, left), and rub the mixture into the skin using soothing, gentle strokes.

• To heal chickenpox lesions, add 2 drops Ravensara, 4 drops Yarrow and 4 drops Lavender to 20g/4 tsp Skin Mousse (see pp.42–3) and apply it as necessary.

Keywords

Invigorating

Supportive

Refreshing

195

Spanish Marjoram (*Thymus mastichina*)

Spanish marjoram is the common name for a plant that looks far more like a kind of thyme than a kind of marjoram – hence the botanical name showing it to be more related to thyme. It has small, pointed, dark-green leaves and produces clusters of tiny white flowers with golden centres. Native to Spain and Portugal, Spanish marjoram makes a pungent herbal tea or inhalation that relieves colds or flu. The essential oil is taken from the flowering tops at the height of summer. It contains a high percentage of eucalyptol, a compound that gives the oil a fresh, sharp and clearing aroma, making it instantly reviving.

Plant features: Low-growing, aromatic herb

Part of plant used: Leaves and flowers

Oil produced in: Spain, Portugal

Extraction method: Steam distillation

Safety first

This oil is non-toxic, non-irritant and non-sensitizing, so is safe for all skin types.

Supporting the spirit

• Spanish Marjoram oil makes the heart feel lighter and opens it to new experiences.
• This essential oil refreshes old thought processes, allowing in bright, new ideas.

Special blends

Add these essential oils to 20ml/4 tsp carrier oil:

To relieve a chesty cough:
4 drops Spanish Marjoram, 4 drops Cardamom, 2 drops Ginger

To ease muscle pain:
4 drops Spanish Marjoram, 4 drops Rosemary, 2 drops Vetiver

Easing the mind

- To help concentration and improve mental focus, vaporize 3 drops Spanish Marjoram and 3 drops Peppermint.
- To relieve mental pressure, take a bath with 2 drops Spanish Marjoram and 4 drops Myrtle.

Healing the body

- To support the body through colds or flu, try an inhalation with 2 drops Spanish Marjoram, 2 drops Black Pepper and 2 drops Lemon.
- To ease chesty coughs and improve breathing, mix Spanish Marjoram with Cardamom and Ginger in a carrier oil (see first blend, left) and rub the blend into your chest every morning and evening.
- To warm and soothe muscular aches and pains, mix Spanish Marjoram with Rosemary and Vetiver in a carrier oil (see second blend, left) and apply the blend to the sore areas twice a day, using long, firm strokes.

Keywords

Clearing

Fresh

Restoring

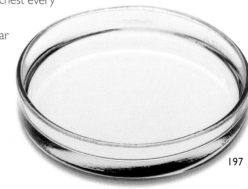

197

Palmarosa *(Cymbopogon martini)*

This tufted grass, which grows wild in northern parts of India, and is now cultivated in the Comoros Islands and the Seychelles, is closely related to Lemongrass (see pp.104–5). In Ayurvedic medicine, the bruised leaves are added to baths to soothe stress. Palmarosa essential oil is used to ease muscle and joint pain, and to relieve nervous tension and fevers. Also an effective insect repellent, this oil has a soft, rosy aroma, with hints of lemon.

Safety first

Palmarosa oil is non-toxic, non-irritating and non-sensitizing, so is safe for all skin types.

Supporting the spirit

- Palmarosa soothes and envelops the heart, protecting against emotional vulnerability.
- This oil calms emotions, bringing inner peace.

Easing the mind

- To ease mental exhaustion and feelings of being overwhelmed, take a bath with 4 drops Palmarosa and 4 drops Mandarin.

Plant features:
Scented tufted grass

Part of plant used:
Leaves

Oil produced in: India, Comoros Islands, Seychelles

Extraction method:
Steam distillation

Special blends

Add these essential oils to 20ml/4 tsp carrier oil:

To even out moods, particularly related to pre-menstrual syndrome (PMS):
4 drops Palmarosa,
4 drops Lemon,
2 drops Neroli

To relieve the physical symptoms of PMS:
4 drops Palmarosa,
4 drops Lavender,
2 drops Vetiver

- To balance mood, mix Palmarosa, Lemon and Neroli in a carrier oil (see first blend, left) and apply, clockwise, to the abdomen twice a day.

Keywords
Subtle
Cooling
Delicate

Healing the body

- To ease the physical symptoms of pre-menstrual syndrome (PMS), such as bloating, mix Palmarosa, Lavender and Vetiver in a carrier oil (see second blend, left) and apply it twice a day in clockwise abdominal strokes.
- To soothe tiredness in the second trimester of pregnancy, take a bath with 2 drops Palmarosa and 2 drops Sweet Orange.
- To tone oily or combination skin, add 4 drops Palmarosa, 4 drops Mandarin and 2 drops Frankincense to 20g/4 tsp Skin Mousse (see pp.42–3) and apply to your face twice a day.
- To repel insects, add 4 drops Palmarosa, 2 drops Patchouli and 4 drops May Chang to 20g/4 tsp Skin Mousse (see pp.42–3) and rub it into exposed areas.

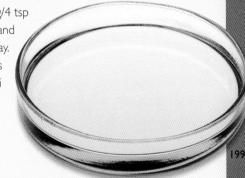

199

Fennel *(Foeniculum vulgare)*

Fennel tea encourages the kidneys to release excess fluid, relieving water retention and making a successful slimming aid. Fennel seeds, when chewed, are a well-known digestive tonic. The oil that comes from the seeds is a mild oestrogen stimulant, so is helpful for menstrual and menopausal conditions. It has a warm, aniseed-like aroma, with peppery notes.

Plant features: Tall annual herb with umbrella-like flowers

Part of plant used: Seeds

Oil produced in: France, Hungary

Extraction method: Steam distillation

Safety first
- Fennel oil is non-toxic and non-irritant, but it is a mild sensitizer: avoid it on sensitive skin.
- Do not use Fennel oil during pregnancy.

Supporting the spirit
- Fennel oil will give you the strength to take action.
- This oil improves stamina to follow a chosen path.

Easing the mind
- To encourage positive thinking, vaporize 3 drops Fennel and 3 drops Sweet Orange.

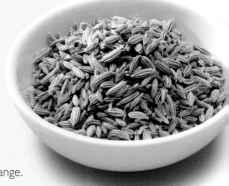

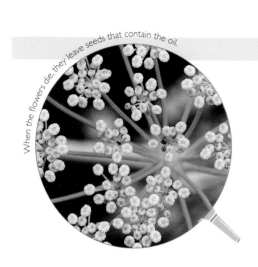

When the flowers die, they leave seeds that contain the oil.

Keywords

Restorative

Balancing

Comforting

- To balance mood swings, take a bath with 2 drops Fennel and 4 drops Palmarosa.

Healing the body
- To regulate periods, mix Fennel, Rose Otto and Bergamot in a carrier oil (see first blend, right) and apply it to the abdomen twice daily.
- To relieve hot flashes, mix Fennel with Agnus Castus and Lavender in a carrier (see second blend, right) and massage it clockwise into the abdomen, chest and shoulders nightly.
- To clarify oily or mature skin, add 4 drops Fennel, 4 drops Frankincense and 2 drops Rose Absolute to 20g/4 tsp Skin Mousse (see pp.42–3) and apply it to your face nightly.

Special blends

Add these essential oils to 20ml/4 tsp carrier oil:

To even out the menstrual cycle:
4 drops Fennel, 2 drops Rose Otto, 4 drops Bergamot

To ease the symptoms of the menopause:
4 drops Fennel, 2 drops Agnus Castus, 4 drops Lavender

Juniper Berry *(Juniperus communis)*

Found in central Europe, the juniper bush produces green buds that, over a period of about two years, gradually mature into black berries. Although famous for making gin, juniper berries are also renowned in Western herbal medicine as one of the most diuretic and detoxifying of all remedies, with a powerful effect on the kidneys. For aromatherapy, always choose Juniper *Berry* essential oil (there is an inferior oil made from twigs). Pungent, woody and peppery, with pine overtones, Juniper Berry is one of the most powerful essential oils available for aromatherapy treatment.

Safety first

- Juniper Berry oil is non-toxic, non-irritating and non-sensitizing, so is safe for all skin types.
- Do not use this oil if you are pregnant.

Supporting the spirit

- Juniper Berry invigorates the heart, promoting inner courage.
- This essential oil protects against negative external influences.

Plant features: Vigorous, evergreen, prickly shrub

Part of plant used: Ripe berries

Oil produced in: Hungary, Croatia

Extraction method: Steam distillation

Special blends

Add these essential oils to 20ml/4 tsp carrier oil:

To ease the physical symptoms of PMS:
2 drops Juniper Berry,
4 drops Grapefruit,
4 drops Fennel

To balance irregular menstrual periods:
2 drops Juniper Berry,
2 drops Agnus Castus,
6 drops Clary Sage

Easing the mind

- To transform mental anxiety and weakness into clarity and strength, vaporize 3 drops Juniper Berry and 3 drops Rosemary.
- To purify negative thoughts and overcome a lack of self-love, take a bath in 2 drops Juniper Berry and 2 drops Rose Absolute.

Healing the body

- To ease the symptoms of pre-menstrual syndrome (PMS), such as water retention, mix Juniper Berry with Grapefruit and Fennel in a carrier oil (see first blend, left) and rub the blend into any areas that are bloated.
- To help to regulate the menstrual cycle, mix Juniper Berry with Agnus Castus and Clary Sage in a carrier oil (see second blend, left) and massage it into the abdomen, using clockwise, circular strokes, every evening.
- To soothe aching muscles, take a bath with 2 drops Juniper Berry and 4 drops Cardamom.

Keywords

Purifying

Invigorating

Cleansing

Sweet Marjoram (*Origanum marjorana*)

This low-growing herb, with small, dark green leaves, and pinkish-white clusters of flowers in midsummer, is a type of oregano, which is native to the southern Mediterranean. In the 17th century, the English herbalist Nicholas Culpeper recommended sweet marjoram for menstrual problems. The fragrance of the essential oil is soft, warm and herbaceous, with woody and slightly spicy undertones.

Safety first

Sweet Marjoram oil is non-toxic, non-irritating and non-sensitizing, so is safe for all skin types.

Supporting the spirit

• Sweet Marjoram is comforting and soothing during times of emotional turbulence.
• This oil encourages safety and inner peace.

Easing the mind

• To calm mood swings and even out erratic emotions, take a bath with 4 drops Sweet Marjoram and 2 drops Australian Sandalwood.

Plant features: Aromatic herb with velvety leaves

Part of plant used: Leaves and flowers

Oil produced in: Egypt, Turkey

Extraction method: Steam distillation

Special blends

Add these essential oils to 20ml/4 tsp carrier oil:

To nurture the spirit during emotional stress:
4 drops Sweet Marjoram, 4 drops Linaloe Wood, 2 drops Neroli

To ease period pain:
4 drops Sweet Marjoram, 2 drops Valerian, 4 drops Lavender

• To provide emotional and
mental support during times
of stress, mix Sweet Marjoram
with Linaloe Wood and Neroli
in a carrier oil (see first blend,
left) and massage into the body
whenever you need a boost.

Healing the body

• To ease menstrual cramps and
related exhaustion, mix Sweet
Marjoram with Valerian and Lavender
in a carrier oil (see second blend, left) and
massage it into the abdomen, using clockwise,
circular strokes, twice a day. Place a hot-water
bottle on your abdomen immediately after
the massage to enhance the effects.

• To soothe deeply aching and tired muscles,
take a bath with 4 drops Sweet Marjoram
and 2 drops Vetiver.

• To soothe headaches or migraines, add
2 drops Sweet Marjoram to 5ml/1 tsp carrier
oil and, using your fingertips, massage the
blend into your forehead.

Keywords

Nurturing

Soothing

Enveloping

205

Clary Sage *(Salvia sclarea)*

This amazing plant is the giant of the sages, growing up to 1.5m/5 ft tall. In midsummer, the plant produces tall spikes of lilac-and-pink flowers that have an incredibly musky aroma. The flowers are so sticky with fragrance that, if you touch them, the essential oil clings to your skin. Musky, nutty and woody-sweet, Clary Sage is one of the most valuable oils for menstrual problems, childbirth and the menopause.

Plant features: Tall herb with aromatic flowers

Part of plant used: Flowering tops

Oil produced in: France

Extraction method: Steam distillation

Safety first

- Clary Sage oil is non-toxic, non-irritant and non-sensitizing, so is safe for all skin types.
- Avoid Clary Sage during pregnancy, although you can use it in labour.

Supporting the spirit

- Clary Sage oil improves a woman's experience of the transitions in her life – puberty, motherhood, and so on.
- This oil symbolizes the "sacred feminine".

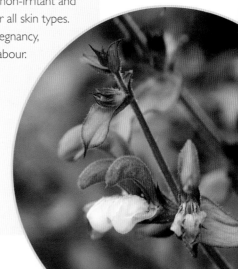

Easing the mind

- To relieve mood swings, take a bath with 2 drops Clary Sage and 4 drops Tangerine.
- To raise low sexual energy, mix Clary Sage with Jasmine Absolute and Australian Sandalwood in a carrier (see first blend, right), and apply to the body using soothing strokes.

Healing the body

- To balance female hormones, blend Clary Sage, Agnus Castus and Rose Geranium in a carrier oil (see second blend, right) and apply it using clockwise abdominal massage.
- To help bring on labour contractions and to feel more calm during childbirth, dilute 2 drops Clary Sage and 2 drops Jasmine Absolute in 20ml/4 tsp carrier oil, and ask your birthing partner to massage the blend into your abdomen and lower back.
- To normalize oily or combination skin, add 2 drops Clary Sage, 4 drops Geranium and 4 drops Mandarin to 20g/4 tsp Skin Mousse (see pp.42–3) and apply the blend to your face nightly.

Keywords

Mood-enhancing

Supportive

Regulating

Special blends

Add these essential oils to 20ml/4 tsp carrier oil:

To boost sexual energy:
4 drops Clary Sage,
2 drops Jasmine Absolute, 4 drops Australian Sandalwood

To regulate periods and balance hormones during the menopause:
4 drops Clary Sage,
2 drops Agnus Castus,
4 drops Rose Geranium

207

Australian Sandalwood (*Santalum spicatum*)

Native to Western Australia, this small tree with aromatic wood has been used to make incense since the 19th century. The tree is now used as a sustainable alternative to Indian sandalwood, which has been overforested, limiting the supply of its essential oil (see box, p.17). The essential oil from Australian sandalwood has a similar aroma to Indian Sandalwood, but is lighter, softer and sweeter, with woody notes.

Plant features: Small tree with fragrant heartwood

Part of plant used: Heartwood

Oil produced in: Australia

Extraction method: Steam distillation

Safety first

Australian Sandalwood oil is non-toxic, non-irritating and non-sensitizing, so is safe for all skin types.

Supporting the spirit

- Australian Sandalwood oil warms and envelops the heart, lessening feelings of vulnerability.
- This oil fortifies an inner resolve to persevere through emotional challenges.

208

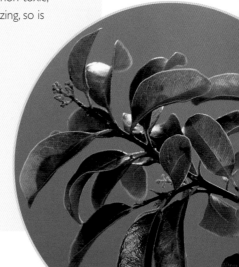

Easing the mind

- To ease mental stress and burnout, take a bath with 2 drops Australian Sandalwood and 4 drops Lavender.
- To calm erratic emotions and hormonal mood swings, mix Australian Sandalwood with Rose Geranium and Clary Sage in a carrier oil (see first blend, right) and apply it with gentle strokes anywhere on your body.

Healing the body

- To ease tiredness, bloating and other physical symptoms of pre-menstrual syndrome (PMS), mix Australian Sandalwood with Fennel and Mandarin in a carrier oil (see second blend, right) and apply it to the appropriate areas.
- To ease backache after six months of pregnancy, take a bath with 2 drops Australian Sandalwood and 2 drops Palmarosa.
- To nourish and regenerate dry or mature skin, add 2 drops Australian Sandalwood, 4 drops Neroli and 4 drops Frankincense to 20g/4 tsp Skin Mousse (see pp.42–3) and apply the blend nightly to your face.

Keywords

Nurturing

Warming

Comforting

Special blends

Add these essential oils to 20ml/4 tsp carrier oil:

To even out moods:
2 drops Australian Sandalwood, 4 drops Rose Geranium, 4 drops Clary Sage

To relieve the physical effects of PMS:
2 drops Australian Sandalwood, 4 drops Fennel, 4 drops Mandarin

209

Agnus Castus (*Vitex agnus castus*)

The name agnus castus means "chaste lamb", a reference to the ancient use of the herb to encourage sexual abstinence in people leading a religious life. Modern research has highlighted the beneficial effects of this plant as a female hormone-enhancer. Although agnus castus is well known in herbalism, the essential oil (from the berries) is fairly new to aromatherapy. It has a very warming, pungent and earthy aroma.

Safety first
- Agnus Castus oil is non-toxic, non-irritating and non-sensitizing, so is safe for all skin types.
- Do not use Agnus Castus during pregnancy.

Supporting the spirit
- Agnus Castus essential oil harnesses and enhances inner feminine energy.
- This essential oil supports the expression of innermost feelings.

Easing the mind
- To calm emotional stress, bathe with 2 drops Agnus Castus and 4 drops Linaloe Wood.

Plant features: Fragrant shrub with pinkish flowers

Part of plant used: Berries

Oil produced in: Crete

Extraction method: Steam distillation

Special blends

Add these essential oils to 20ml/4 tsp carrier oil:

To even out moods and relieve sadness:
2 drops Agnus Castus, 2 drops Vetiver, 6 drops Australian Sandalwood

To regulate hormones during menstruation or the menopause:
2 drops Agnus Castus, 4 drops Clary Sage, 4 drops Geranium

• To calm mood swings and tearfulness, mix Agnus Castus with Vetiver and Australian Sandalwood in a carrier (see first blend, left) and apply the blend to your body in any way that feels supportive.

Healing the body

• To regulate menstruation or to balance hormones in early menopause, apply Agnus Castus with Clary Sage and Geranium in a carrier oil (see second blend, left), using clockwise abdominal massage.

• To ease headaches and physical exhaustion resulting from pre-menstrual syndrome (PMS), take a bath with 2 drops Agnus Castus and 2 drops Rose Absolute.

• This oil is said to boost female fertility. Dilute 4 drops Agnus Castus, 2 drops Vetiver and 4 drops Rose Otto in 20ml/4 tsp carrier and ask your partner to massage the blend into your back and/or abdomen once or twice a week, especially around the time of ovulation.

Keywords
Feminine
Pungent
Grounding

Citronella (Cymbopogon nardus)

Native to Sri Lanka, this lemon-scented grass is a close relative of lemongrass (see pp.104–5) and palmarosa (see pp.198–9). In Sri Lankan local medicine, crushed leaves were once used to heal wounds. In the West, citronella (which is rich in the biochemical ingredient citronellal) is best known as an insect repellent. The oil has a soft and sweet lemony aroma.

Plant features:
Tufted aromatic grass

Part of plant used:
Leaves

Oil produced in:
Sri Lanka

Extraction method:
Steam distillation

Safety first
• Citronella oil is non-toxic.
• This oil can be a moderate irritant and sensitizer: avoid it in baths or massage if you have sensitive or allergy-prone skin.

Supporting the spirit
• Citronella provides gentle nurturing during periods of self-doubt.
• This essential oil lightens heavy emotional burdens and encourages hopefulness.

Easing the mind
• To ease anxiety, sadness or depression, blend Citronella with Neroli and Australian

Special blends

Add these essential oils to 20ml/4 tsp carrier oil:

To lift the spirits and relieve anxiety:
4 drops Citronella,
2 drops Neroli, 4 drops
Australian Sandalwood

To enable clear thinking:
4 drops Citronella,
2 drops Patchouli,
4 drops Bergamot Mint

Sandalwood in a carrier oil (see first blend, left) and rub it into your neck and shoulders.

- To lift confusion and relieve stress, helping you to see a clear path, mix Citronella with Patchouli and Bergamot Mint in a carrier oil (see second blend, left) and gently rub the blend into the areas where you store tension.

Healing the body

- To ease physical exhaustion, take a bath with 2 drops Citronella and 4 drops Myrtle.
- To soothe indigestion and boost a sluggish digestive system, dilute 4 drops Citronella and 6 drops Spearmint in 20ml/4 tsp carrier oil and apply the blend to your abdomen twice a day, using gentle, clockwise strokes.
- To keep mosquitoes at bay, add 4 drops Citronella, 2 drops Patchouli and 4 drops Himalayan Cedarwood to 20g/4 tsp Skin Mousse (see pp.42–3) and apply it as an insect repellent to exposed areas of skin.

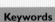

Keywords
Light
Soft
Clarifying

213

May Chang *(Litsea cubeba)*

The name may chang is an anglicized spelling of the Chinese name meaning "mountain spicy tree". The tree has delicate foliage and flowers, and produces small fruit that resemble cubeb seeds (pp. 174–5), hence its Latin name. Traditional Chinese Medicine uses may chang fruit to ease digestive complaints, as well as to relieve lower-back pain and muscular stiffness. Research has shown that the fruit, which yields the essential oil, also helps to regulate blood pressure. The oil is rich in citral, a compound with a fizzy, zesty lemon aroma, which becomes sweeter and softer as the oil evaporates.

Safety first
- May Chang oil is non-toxic.
- This essential oil can be a moderate skin irritant or sensitizer: avoid it in baths or massage if you have sensitive skin.

Supporting the spirit
- May Chang creates a sense of inner lightness.
- This oil dissolves chronic negative emotional patterns and will enable a fresh start.

Plant features: Tropical tree with delicate leaves

Part of plant used: Peppercorn-like fruit

Oil produced in: China

Extraction method: Steam distillation

Special blends

Add these essential oils to 20ml/4 tsp carrier oil:

To relieve stress:
2 drops May Chang,
4 drops Rose Otto,
4 drops Roman Chamomile

To lift depression and improve mood:
2 drops May Chang,
4 drops Neroli, 4 drops Orange Leaf

Easing the mind

- To calm anxiety, mix May Chang with Rose Otto and Roman Chamomile in a carrier oil (see first blend, left) and ask a partner to massage the blend into your back.
- To lighten heavy moods, mix May Chang with Neroli and Orange Leaf in a carrier oil (see second blend, left) and gently rub the blend into your upper body, concentrating on the chest, neck and shoulders.
- To improve concentration, vaporize 3 drops May Chang and 3 drops Peppermint.

Healing the body

- To support the body's systems through post-viral fatigue, take a bath with 2 drops May Chang and 4 drops Cardamom.
- To ease indigestion, blend 2 drops May Chang, 4 drops Peppermint and 4 drops Ginger in 20ml/4 tsp carrier oil and apply it using clockwise abdominal strokes, twice a day.

Keywords
Revitalizing
Zesty
Sweet

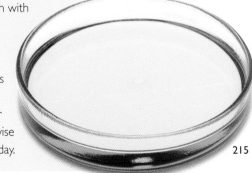

215

Nutmeg *(Myristica fragans)*

When nutmegs first appeared in medieval Europe, they were so valuable that they were often carried about in small, locked boxes, chained to people's girdles. Sprinkled over a hot milky drink, they were believed to allay nightmares and give good rest. Across Indonesia and Malaysia, where nutmeg trees are native, the oil is valued as a painkilling remedy. It has a fresh, sharp and sweet aroma, becoming rich, warm and spicy as the oil evaporates.

Plant features: Tropical tree producing aromatic fruit

Part of plant used:
Seeds (nutmegs)

Oil produced in:
Indonesia, Malaysia

Extraction method:
Steam distillation

Safety first
Nutmeg essential oil is non-toxic, non-irritating and non-sensitizing, so is safe for all skin types.

Supporting the spirit
• Nutmeg dissolves fear and
  promotes self-confidence.
• This oil will alleviate sadness
  and bring brighter moods.

Easing the mind
• To lift depression, anxiety or low self-esteem,
  mix Nutmeg with May Chang and Neroli in

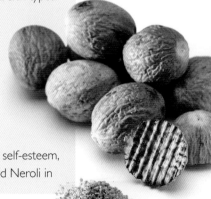

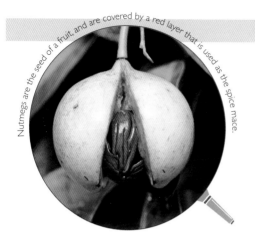

Nutmegs are the seed of a fruit, and are covered by a red layer that is used as the spice mace.

Keywords
Cheering
Fortifying
Refreshing

a carrier oil (see first blend, right) and apply it to your skin with soothing strokes.

- To even out mood swings, vaporize 2 drops Nutmeg and 4 drops Grapefruit.
- To overcome insomnia, mix Nutmeg with Lavender and Linaloe Wood in a carrier (see second blend, right) and gently rub the blend into your neck and shoulders each evening.

Healing the body

- To ease muscular aches and pains, bathe with 2 drops Nutmeg and 4 drops Linaloe Wood.
- To calm indigestion, blend 2 drops Nutmeg, 4 drops Coriander Seed and 4 drops Ginger in 20ml/4 tsp carrier and apply to the abdomen.

Special blends

Add these essential oils to 20ml/4 tsp carrier oil:

To improve low moods and lift anxiety:
2 drops Nutmeg,
4 drops May Chang,
4 drops Neroli

To aid restful sleep:
2 drops Nutmeg,
4 drops Lavender,
4 drops Linaloe Wood

217

Sweet Basil *(Ocimum basilicum)*

Different species of basil are found all over the world, but this is the Mediterranean basil, which thrives in hot, dry, sunny climates and is famously used in Italian cooking. The plant produces lush, highly aromatic green leaves, with tall spikes of white flowers at the end of summer. The essential oil is strongest in the leaves before the plant flowers. The 17th-century English herbalist Nicholas Culpeper recommended sweet basil to treat insect and snake bites. The oil has a fresh and herbaceous aroma, with rich, warm, spicy undertones.

Plant features: Aromatic herb with lush green leaves

Part of plant used: Leaves

Oil produced in: Egypt

Extraction method: Steam distillation

Safety first
- Sweet Basil oil is non-sensitizing and non-toxic in low concentrations.
- This oil can be a mild irritant: avoid it in baths or massage if you have delicate skin.
- Do not use Sweet Basil during pregnancy.

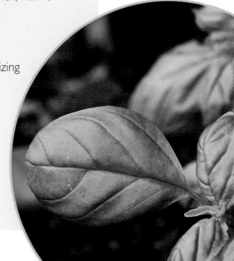

Supporting the spirit
• Sweet Basil enhances courage and gives you the energy to tackle new experiences.
• This oil clarifies inner goals.

Easing the mind
• To relieve anxiety and mental overload, mix Sweet Basil, Lavender and Australian Sandalwood in a carrier oil (see first blend, right) and rub it into your neck and shoulders.
• To improve concentration, vaporize 2 drops Sweet Basil and 4 drops Myrtle.
• To ease emotional vulnerability, mix Sweet Basil with Sweet Orange and Orange Leaf in a carrier oil (see second blend, right) and smooth it into your skin as appropriate.

Healing the body
• To settle nervous digestive upsets, bathe with 2 drops Sweet Basil and 4 drops Orange Leaf.
• To heal insect bites and stings, mix 2 drops Sweet Basil, 4 drops Tea Tree and 4 drops Manuka in 20g/4 tsp Skin Mousse (see pp.42–3) and apply it to the affected area.

Keywords
Warm
Fiery
Strengthening

Special blends

Add these essential oils to 20ml/4 tsp carrier oil:

To lift anxiety or calm an overactive mind:
2 drops Sweet Basil,
4 drops Lavender,
4 drops Australian Sandalwood

To relieve feelings of emotional fragility:
2 drops Sweet Basil,
4 drops Sweet Orange,
4 drops Orange Leaf

219

Tulsi (*Ocimum sanctum*)

In India, tulsi is a holy plant sacred to the goddess Vrindavani – beloved of Lord Vishnu, the supreme deity of the Indian pantheon. Also known as Indian Holy Basil, it is used as a cooking herb, rubbed on the skin to keep away mosquitoes and drunk as *jushanda*, an infusion to ease bronchitis, colds and flu. Indian holy men, called Brahmins, have leaves of tulsi placed on their faces, eyes, ears and chest when they die and pass into the next world. The essential oil has a strong fragrance, from a spicy ingredient called eugenol (which is also present in Clove Bud). Tulsi also has fresh, sweet notes as it evaporates.

Plant features: Aromatic herb with lush foliage

Part of plant used: Leaves

Oil produced in: India

Extraction method: Steam distillation

Safety first

- Tulsi oil is non-toxic in low doses, but it can be a mild irritant or sensitizer: avoid it in baths or massage for sensitive skin.
- Do not use Tulsi oil during pregnancy.

220

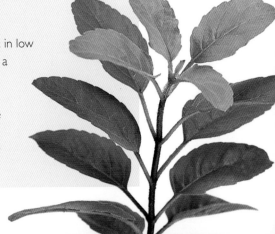

Supporting the spirit

- Tulsi opens the heart in readiness to receive the love of your soulmate.
- This oil strengthens a sense of inner purpose, enabling you to focus on new possibilities.

Easing the mind

- To lift mental exhaustion and renew zest for life, mix Tulsi with Neroli and Linaloe Wood in a carrier oil (see first blend, right) and massage it into the neck and shoulders.
- To soothe anxiety and emotional stress, vaporize 2 drops Tulsi and 4 drops Mandarin.
- To take the mind to a place of inner peace, mix Tulsi with Frankincense and Himalayan Cedarwood in a carrier oil (see second blend, right) and apply it wherever feels soothing.

Healing the body

- To help the body through colds and flu, bathe with 2 drops Tulsi and 4 drops Cardamom.
- To ease coughs, bronchitis or laryngitis, try a regular inhalation with 2 drops Tulsi and 2 drops Black Cumin Seed.

Keywords

Embracing

Warming

Comforting

Special blends

Add these essential oils to 20ml/4 tsp carrier oil:

To relieve a tired mind:
2 drops Tulsi, 4 drops Neroli, 4 drops Linaloe Wood

To bring deep peace and relaxation:
2 drops Tulsi, 4 drops Frankincense, 4 drops Himalayan Cedarwood

221

Damiana *(Turnera diffusa)*

Found mainly in Mexico and the West Indies, the damiana plant has vivid green, serrated leaves and golden yellow flowers that die to leave pungent-smelling seeds. In Mexican herbal medicine, damiana is a nerve and reproductive tonic for both sexes. Legend has it that the Aztecs and Mayans drank its infusion to enhance fertility. Damiana essential oil is rare and available only from specialist suppliers who are in contact with growers. It has a complex aroma, with warm, woody-sweet and spicy notes.

Safety first
- Damiana oil is non-toxic, non-irritant and non-sensitizing, so is safe for all skin types.
- Do not use Damiana during pregnancy, as it is a powerful menstrual stimulant.

Supporting the spirit
- Damiana essential oil strengthens and helps to maintain inner vitality.
- This essential oil lessens emotional instability owing to its grounding and calming effects.

Plant features: Shrub with serrated leaves and yellow flowers

Part of plant used: Leaves

Oil produced in: Mexico, West Indies

Extraction method: Steam distillation

Special blends

Add these essential oils to 20ml/4 tsp carrier oil:

To relieve ongoing or recurrent stress:
2 drops Damiana, 4 drops Neroli, 4 drops Australian Sandalwood

To renew sexual energy and improve fertility:
2 drops Damiana, 6 drops Cardamom, 2 drops Jasmine Absolute

Easing the mind

- To soothe chronic stress and hypersensitivity, mix Damiana with Neroli and Australian Sandalwood in a carrier oil (see first blend, left); massage it into the neck and shoulders.
- To calm overstretched nerves, bathe with 2 drops Damiana and 4 drops Orange Leaf.
- To soothe anxieties, especially over fertility issues, dilute 2 drops Damiana, 6 drops Rose Geranium and 2 drops Vetiver in 20ml/4 tsp carrier oil and apply it to the abdomen in clockwise strokes.

Healing the body

- To regenerate sexual energy and improve fertility, mix Damiana with Cardamom and Jasmine Absolute in a carrier oil (see second blend, left) and apply it in clockwise abdominal massage, daily.
- To regulate menstruation and ease menstrual cramping, take a bath with 2 drops Damiana and 4 drops Sweet Marjoram.

Keywords

Regenerating

Restorative

Warming

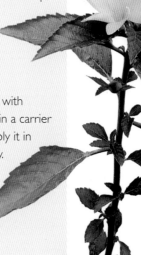

223

Valerian (*Valeriana officinalis*)

One of the oldest remedies in Western herbal medicine to soothe sleep problems and mental stress, valerian is an unscented plant above the ground, but its thick roots beneath the ground are highly pungent. The 17th-century English herbalist Nicholas Culpeper recommended valerian root for "headaches, tremblings, palpitations and hysteric complaints". Modern herbalists use the dried root as a sedative. Valerian essential oil is one of the most powerful-smelling oils, with a musky, heavy and woody scent. You need use only small amounts.

Plant features: Herb with dark green leaves, and pink or white flowers

Part of plant used: Roots

Oil produced in: France, UK

Extraction method: Steam distillation

Safety first
- Valerian oil is non-toxic and non-irritant.
- This oil is a potential sensitizer: avoid it in baths or massage if you have sensitive skin.
- Valerian oil has a deeply sedative effect: do not drive or operate machinery for at least eight hours after using it.

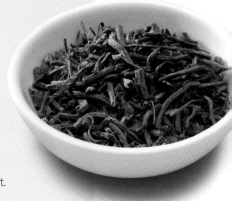

Supporting the spirit

- Valerian oil stabilizes erratic, scattered energy, bringing back a sense of balance to the spirit.
- This essential oil promotes inner tranquillity.

Easing the mind

- To soothe emotional stress and overcome insecurity, mix Valerian with Australian Sandalwood and Laurel Leaf in a carrier oil (see first blend, right) and apply it to the body wherever you find it soothing.
- To overcome panic, mix Valerian with Neroli and May Chang in a carrier oil (see second blend, right) and apply the blend gently to the neck and shoulders.
- To help to combat insomnia, vaporize 2 drops Valerian and 4 drops Himalayan Cedarwood in your bedroom as you go to sleep.

Healing the body

- To ease backache, take a bath with 2 drops Valerian and 4 drops Black Spruce.
- To soothe indigestion, bathe with 2 drops Valerian and 4 drops Ginger.

Keywords

Soothing

Grounding

Powerful

Special blends

Add these essential oils to 20ml/4 tsp carrier oil:

To feel calm and more emotionally secure:
2 drops Valerian, 4 drops Australian Sandalwood, 4 drops Laurel Leaf

To ease away fear and calm panic attacks:
2 drops Valerian, 4 drops Neroli, 4 drops May Chang

225

Angelica Root *(Angelica archangelica)*

A member of the *Umbelliferae* family, which produces umbrella-like flowering heads, angelica's flowers create a kind of "halo" around the stem, perhaps accounting for the Latin name *archangelica*. Angelica Root oil has a clearing aroma, with aniseed and spicy hints.

Plant features: Tall vigorous herb, with spherical flower clusters

Part of plant used: Roots

Oil produced in: Hungary, Belgium

Extraction method: Steam distillation

Safety first
- Angelica Root oil is non-toxic and non-irritant.
- This oil is a mild sensitizer: avoid it in baths or massage if you have sensitive skin.
- This oil is phototoxic: avoid it in baths or massage if you are going out in the sun.
- Avoid Angelica Root during pregnancy.

Supporting the spirit
- Angelica Root enhances awareness of the spirit.
- This oil promotes self-belief.

Easing the mind
- To relieve mental pressure, vaporize 2 drops Angelica Root and 4 drops Grapefruit.

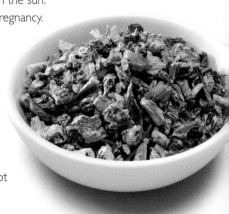

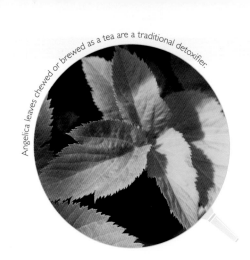

Angelica leaves chewed or brewed as a tea are a traditional detoxifier.

Keywords

Refreshing

Purifying

Cleansing

• To encourage mental stamina during extreme fatigue, take a bath with 2 drops Angelica Root and 4 drops Rose Geranium.

Healing the body

• To ease digestive problems, blend Angelica Root, Ginger and Coriander Seed in a carrier oil (see first blend, right) and apply it in clockwise abdominal strokes, twice daily.

• To detoxify cellulite, apply a blend of Angelica Root, Grapefruit and Juniper Berry in a carrier oil (see second blend, right) to affected areas.

• To soothe rheumatic pain or gout, take a bath with 2 drops Angelica Root and 4 drops Roman Chamomile.

Special blends

Add these essential oils to 20ml/4 tsp carrier oil:

To relieve indigestion or nausea:
2 drops Angelica Root, 4 drops Ginger, 4 drops Coriander Seed

To reduce cellulite and ease water retention:
2 drops Angelica Root, 4 drops Grapefruit, 4 drops Juniper Berry

227

Grapefruit (*Citrus × paradisi*)

Originally cultivated in the West Indies, although now mostly grown in Florida and Brazil, grapefruit are believed to be a cross between a large citrus fruit called a pomelo (*Citrus maximus*) and the sweet orange (*Citrus sinensis*; see pp.232–3). The grapefruit tree has dark, glossy leaves and beautiful white flowers that become the yellow fruit. Like all citrus species, grapefruit contain special sacs in their peel, which are filled with essential oil. Grapefruit essential oil has a green and fresh aroma, with fizzy citrus and fruity top notes.

Safety first
• Grapefruit oil is non-toxic, non-irritant and non-sensitizing, so is safe for all skin types.
• This oil is phototoxic: avoid it in baths or massage if you are going out in the sun.

Supporting the spirit
• Grapefruit relieves heavy emotional burdens, giving a lightness of spirit.
• Grapefruit opens the heart to enable free expression of love and happiness.

Plant features:
Evergreen citrus tree

Part of plant used:
Fruit peel

Oil produced in:
West Indies, US, Brazil

Extraction method:
Expression

Special blends

Add these essential oils to 20ml/4 tsp carrier oil:

To ease the passage of rich food through the system:
4 drops Grapefruit,
4 drops Peppermint,
2 drops Ginger

To aid the removal of toxins from the body:
4 drops Grapefruit,
4 drops Juniper, 2 drops Angelica Root

Easing the mind

- To ease nervous exhaustion, take a bath with
  2 drops Grapefruit and 4 drops Geranium.
- To help to relieve depression and lift dark
  moods, vaporize 4 drops Grapefruit and
  2 drops Frankincense.

Healing the body

- To ease indigestion caused by rich food, or to
  reduce feelings of nausea, mix Grapefruit with
  Peppermint and Ginger in a carrier oil (see
  first blend, left) and apply it using clockwise
  abdominal massage, twice a day.
- To detoxify the body's systems (in particular
  the lymphatic systems and the kidneys)
  and to reduce cellulite, mix Grapefruit with
  Juniper and Angelica Root in a carrier oil (see
  second blend, left) and apply the blend to the
  affected areas (usually the thighs).
- To clarify and tone oily, combination or
  problem skin, add 4 drops Grapefruit,
  2 drops Cypress and 4 drops Myrtle to
  20g/4 tsp Skin Mousse (see pp.42–3) and
  apply it to your face nightly.

Keywords
Revitalizing
Refreshing
Cheering

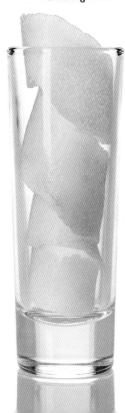

229

Tangerine (*Citrus reticulata* 'Blanco')

Closely related to the mandarin tree (see pp.258–9), the tangerine tree produces cream-coloured flowers and small orange fruit. The tangerine fruit are slightly more oval than mandarins and have paler, yellow-orange peel. Pare off a thin strip of this peel, and you can clearly see that the underside is covered in tiny sacs, which are full of the fruit's essential oil. If you press the peel between your fingers, you will release the oil's beautiful aroma, which is extensively used in the perfumery industry, as well as in aromatherapy. Expressing the oil from the peel preserves all the fresh citrus notes in its fragrance, as well as its bittersweet green hints and subtle sweet notes.

Safety first

- Tangerine oil is non-toxic, non-irritant and non-sensitizing, making it safe for all skin types.
- Tangerine is a sun-safe citrus oil. Unlike many other citrus oils, it is not phototoxic, so you can use it on your skin even when you are planning to go out in the sun.

Plant features: Evergreen tree with cream flowers

Part of plant used: Fruit peel

Oil produced in: US

Extraction method: Expression

Special blends

Add these essential oils to 20ml/4 tsp carrier oil:

To ease cramps or indigestion:
4 drops Tangerine,
2 drops Peppermint,
4 drops Carrot Seed

To improve the appearance of normal, oily or mature skin:
4 drops Tangerine,
2 drops Rose Absolute,
4 drops Frankincense

Supporting the spirit
- Tangerine oil opens the heart to spontaneity.
- This oil reveals a sense of innocence.

Easing the mind
- To relieve depression, vaporize 4 drops Tangerine and 2 drops Geranium.
- To lighten mental overload, take a bath with 4 drops Mandarin and 2 drops Ylang Ylang.

Healing the body
- To soothe digestive discomfort, mix Tangerine with Peppermint and Carrot Seed in a carrier oil (see first blend, left) and apply it to the abdomen using clockwise strokes, twice a day.
- To reduce the appearance of stretch marks, if you are more than five months pregnant, dilute 2 drops Tangerine and 2 drops Neroli in 20ml/4 tsp carrier oil and rub it into the abdomen, in a clockwise direction, daily.
- To tone and clarify normal, oily or mature skin, mix Tangerine with Rose Absolute and Frankincense in a carrier oil (see second blend, left) and apply it to your face nightly.

Keywords

Light

Encouraging

Uplifting

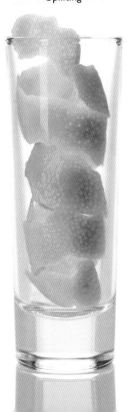

231

Sweet Orange (*Citrus sinensis*)

No-one knows exactly how citrus trees, originally native to southern China, arrived in western Europe, but one theory goes that early Arab or Portuguese traders may have found their way to India, the Himalayas and China, and brought back seeds for cultivation. For hundreds of years, orange trees naturalized themselves in the hot, dry climate of the Mediterranean, and are now cultivated all over the world, especially in Italy and Israel. Sweet Orange essential oil has a light, sweet aroma with soft citrus notes.

Safety first

- Sweet Orange oil is non-toxic, non-irritating and non-sensitizing, so is safe for all skin types.
- Sweet Orange is a sun-safe citrus oil. Unlike many other citrus oils, it is not phototoxic, so you can use it on your skin even if you are planning to go out in the sun.

Supporting the spirit

- Sweet Orange is uplifting for the spirit and helps to brighten moods.

Plant features:
Evergreen citrus tree

Part of plant used:
Fruit peel

Oil produced in:
Italy, Israel

Extraction method:
Expression

Special blends

Add these essential oils to 20ml/4 tsp carrier oil:

To stabilize mood:
4 drops Sweet Orange,
2 drops Rose Absolute,
4 drops Australian
Sandalwood

To improve digestion:
6 drops Sweet Orange,
4 drops Neroli *(This blend is especially suitable for children aged over two if you halve the drops.)*

• This essential oil encourages feelings of joy and happiness deep within.

Easing the mind
• To alleviate anxiety and insomnia, vaporize 4 drops Sweet Orange and 2 drops Myrtle.
• To overcome mood swings and soothe away sadness, mix Sweet Orange with Rose Absolute and Australian Sandalwood in a carrier oil (see first blend, left) and apply it to your body wherever it feels comforting.

Healing the body
• To ease indigestion and constipation, mix Sweet Orange with Neroli (see second blend, left) and apply it to the abdomen using circular, clockwise strokes, twice daily.
• To soothe tiredness after six months of pregnancy, take a bath with 2 drops Sweet Orange and 2 drops Linaloe Wood.
• To unclog pores in oily or combination skin, add 4 drops Sweet Orange, 2 drops Cypress and 4 drops Orange Leaf to 20g/4 tsp Skin Mousse (see pp.42–3) and apply to your face.

Keywords

Gentle

Nurturing

Sweet

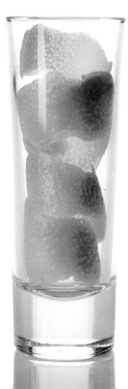

233

Coriander Seed *(Coriandrum sativum)*

A well-known digestive tonic, the coriander plant is a member of the *Umbelliferae* botanical family – it produces clusters of flowers on splayed stalks, called "umbels". Once dead, these blooms leave behind essential-oil-rich seeds. In China, coriander seeds have been chewed for centuries to sweeten the breath and promote a long life. Pleasant-smelling, with a woody, spicy fragrance and soft, sweet notes, Coriander Seed essential oil is milder than many other spice oils, with a gentle effect on both body and mind.

Plant features: Aromatic herb with umbel flowers

Part of plant used: Seeds

Oil produced in: France

Extraction method: Steam distillation

Safety first

Coriander Seed oil is non-toxic, non-irritating and non-sensitizing, so is safe for all skin types.

Supporting the spirit

- This oil gently supports and nurtures the "inner child".
- Coriander Seed essential oil helps to promote a positive outlook and foster new ideas.

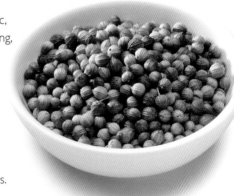

Easing the mind

- To ease mental stress and nervous tension, take a bath with 4 drops Coriander Seed and 2 drops Sweet Orange.
- To ease away insomnia caused by mental stress, vaporize 3 drops Coriander Seed and 3 drops Australian Sandalwood.

Healing the body

- To ease constipation, sluggish digestion or indigestion caused by nervousness or stress, mix Coriander Seed with Spearmint and Neroli in a carrier oil (see first blend, right) and rub the blend into your abdomen, using clockwise strokes, twice a day.
- To support the body's systems through post-viral fatigue, mix Coriander Seed with Cubeb Seed and Patchouli in a carrier oil (see second blend, right) and apply the blend gently to your body as necessary, wherever it feels most soothing to do so.
- To boost poor circulation and ease muscular stiffness, take a bath with 4 drops Coriander Seed and 2 drops Cardamom.

Keywords

Calming

Soft

Warming

Special blends

Add these essential oils to 20ml/4 tsp carrier oil:

To treat constipation and boost digestion:
4 drops Coriander Seed,
4 drops Spearmint,
2 drops Neroli

To speed the body's recovery from viruses:
4 drops Coriander Seed,
4 drops Cubeb Seed,
2 drops Patchouli

235

Turmeric (*Curcuma longa*)

Like its relatives ginger (see pp.120–21) and plai (see pp.118–19), turmeric contains its aroma in its root tissue, perhaps to ward off burrowing insects. In Ayurvedic medicine, turmeric root is used as an all-round internal cleanser, as well as a digestive and urinary tonic. Modern research shows that, eaten regularly, the spice may reduce the risk of contracting bowel cancer. The oil has a gentle, warm, spicy aroma, with earthy subtle notes.

Safety first
Turmeric oil is non-toxic, non-irritating and non-sensitizing, so is safe for all skin types.

Supporting the spirit
• Turmeric essential oil gently grounds a flighty spirit and centres scattered energy.
• This essential oil strengthens inner confidence and provides the resolve to take action.

Easing the mind
• To calm anger and fiery emotions, bathe with 2 drops Turmeric and 4 drops Bergamot Mint.

Plant features: Tropical plant with fleshy root

Part of plant used: Roots

Oil produced in: India

Extraction method: Steam distillation

Special blends

Add these essential oils to 20ml/4 tsp carrier oil:

To ease the bowel and combat indigestion:
4 drops Turmeric,
4 drops Nutmeg,
2 drops Cardamom

To support the body through chronic exhaustion:
4 drops Turmeric,
4 drops Bergamot,
2 drops Neroli

- To soothe mental stress, vaporize 2 drops Turmeric and 4 drops Mandarin.

Healing the body

- To ease the symptoms of irritable bowel syndrome or nervous indigestion, mix Turmeric with Nutmeg and Cardamom in a carrier oil (see first blend, left) and apply using clockwise abdominal massage, twice a day.
- To support the body through chronic fatigue or post-viral conditions, mix Turmeric with Bergamot and Neroli in a carrier oil (see second blend, left) and use the blend to give yourself a gentle, soothing massage.
- To ease backache or rheumatic pain, take a bath with 4 drops Turmeric and 2 drops Vetiver.
- To heal wounds, cuts and sores, add 4 drops Turmeric, 2 drops German Chamomile and 4 drops Lavender to 20g/4 tsp Skin Mousse (see pp.42–3) and apply it to the affected areas.

Keywords

Cleansing

Balancing

Warming

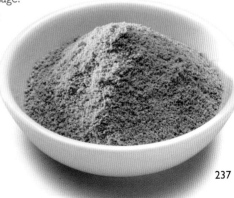

237

Carrot Seed *(Daucus carota)*

Found throughout northern Europe, the wild carrot has erect, hairy stems and odourless leaves, and produces flat umbels of tiny white flowers in late summer. These die back, leaving a "head" of pungent seeds, which have been used for hundreds of years as a digestive tonic. The 17th-century English herbalist Nicholas Culpeper recommended them for colicky pains and wind. In modern Western herbal medicine, carrot seed powder is used to ease fluid retention and indigestion. The essential oil from the seeds is musty, earthy and subtle, with woody notes as it evaporates.

Safety first

Carrot Seed essential oil is non-toxic, non-irritating and non-sensitizing, making it suitable for all skin types.

Supporting the spirit

- Carrot Seed warms and supports, easing away feelings of fragility and vulnerability.
- This essential oil creates a sense of inner peace and security.

Plant features: Wild herb with white flowers

Part of plant used: Seeds

Oil produced in: France

Extraction method: Steam distillation

Special blends

Add these essential oils to 20ml/4 tsp carrier oil:

To ease digestive pain or discomfort:
4 drops Carrot Seed, 2 drops Fennel, 4 drops Grapefruit

To relieve water retention and PMS:
4 drops Carrot Seed, 4 drops Lemon, 2 drops Geranium

Easing the mind

- To help insomnia, especially when the mind cannot switch off, vaporize 3 drops Carrot Seed and 3 drops Lavender in your room as you go to bed.
- To soothe chronic emotional stress, enabling deep relaxation, take a bath with 2 drops Carrot Seed and 4 drops Rose Geranium.

Healing the body

- To soothe colic, digestive cramps or irritable bowel syndrome, mix Carrot Seed, Fennel and Grapefruit in a carrier oil (see first blend, left) and apply in clockwise abdominal strokes.
- To relieve the symptoms of pre-menstrual syndrome (PMS), mix Carrot Seed with Lemon and Geranium in a carrier (see second blend, left) and rub into the abdomen.
- To replenish dry or mature skin, add 4 drops Carrot Seed, 2 drops Rose Otto and 4 drops Frankincense to 20g/4 tsp Skin Mousse (see pp.42–3) and apply it to your face nightly.

Keywords
Calming
Restorative
Supportive

239

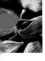

Cardamom (*Elettaria cardamomum*)

Unlike its relatives plai (see pp.118–19), ginger (see pp.120–21) and turmeric (see pp.236–7), cardamom does not have aromatic roots. Its fragrance is concentrated in its pods, which contain the small, dark brown, pungent seeds that provide cardamom's therapeutic essential oil. In Ayurvedic medicine, the seeds are boiled in milk or made into a tea to help the body through viruses; they are also used to stimulate the digestion. A tonic to the body and mind, Cardamom oil has a mouthwatering aroma – sweet and warm, with rich, spicy notes.

Plant features: Tropical plant with cream and purple flowers

Part of plant used: Seeds

Oil produced in: India

Extraction method: Steam distillation

Safety first

Cardamom oil is non-toxic, non-irritating and non-sensitizing, so is safe for all skin types.

Supporting the spirit

- Cardamom gives strength to act on decisions.
- This essential oil encourages a spirit of adventure, helping you to look to new horizons.

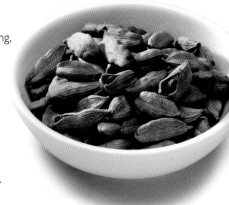

Easing the mind

- To improve concentration and memory recall, vaporize 3 drops Cardamom and 3 drops Cinnamon Leaf.
- To energize and refresh an uninspired, lethargic mind, take a bath with 2 drops Cardamom and 4 drops Mandarin.

Healing the body

- To ease indigestion or stomach cramps, mix Cardamom with Ginger and Sweet Orange in a carrier oil (see first blend, right) and apply it using clockwise abdominal massage as often as necessary until symptoms subside.
- To soothe chronic respiratory problems, as well as coughs and chest infections, mix Cardamom with Himalayan Cedarwood and Benzoin Resinoid in a carrier oil (see second blend, right) and rub it into the chest, twice a day.
- To support the body's systems through viral infections, speeding recovery, try inhalations and a daily bath containing 2 drops Cardamom and 4 drops Bergamot.

Keywords

Fiery

Sweet

Strengthening

Special blends

Add these essential oils to 20ml/4 tsp carrier oil:

To relieve stomach discomfort or pain:
2 drops Cardamom,
2 drops Ginger,
4 drops Sweet Orange

To ease ongoing respiratory illness:
4 drops Cardamom,
4 drops Himalayan Cedarwood, 2 drops Benzoin Resinoid

241

Lovage Root (*Levisticum officinale*)

An important remedy in Western herbal medicine, the lovage plant (all of which is aromatic) has powerful diuretic and detoxifying effects. In his 17th-century text *The Complete Herbal*, Nicholas Culpeper said that the root "provokes urine, ... warms a cold stomach, helps digestion". The oil from the root is warm, spicy and sweet with deep, earthy notes. It is very pungent and powerful so you need to use only small amounts in aromatherapy.

Safety first
- Lovage Root oil is non-toxic and non-irritant.
- This oil is a skin sensitizer: avoid it in baths or massage if you have sensitive skin.
- Lovage Root is phototoxic: avoid it in baths or massage if you are going out in the sun.
- Do not use Lovage Root during pregnancy.

Supporting the spirit
- Lovage Root comforts you if you feel sad and will nurture you back to contentment.
- This essential oil provides a security blanket against others' negativity or anger.

Plant features: Vigorous aromatic herb

Part of plant used: Roots

Oil produced in: Hungary

Extraction method: Steam distillation

Special blends

Add these essential oils to 20ml/4 tsp carrier oil:

To ease digestive problems:
1 drop Lovage Root,
4 drops Peppermint,
4 drops Ginger

To balance the menstrual cycle:
1 drop Lovage Root,
4 drops Damiana,
4 drops Fennel

Easing the mind

- To ease mental stress resulting in digestive upsets, vaporize 1 drop Lovage Root and 4 drops Peppermint.
- To soothe fiery emotions, bathe with 1 drop Lovage Root and 4 drops Orange Leaf.

Healing the body

- To ease indigestion or wind, or tension in the abdomen, mix Lovage Root with Peppermint and Ginger in a carrier oil (see first blend, left) and apply the blend using clockwise abdominal strokes, twice a day.
- To soothe rheumatic or arthritic pain, take a bath with 1 drop Lovage Root and 3 drops Vetiver.
- To regulate erratic menstrual periods, mix Lovage Root with Damiana and Fennel in a carrier oil (see second blend, left) and apply it to the abdomen using clockwise strokes, every evening during your cycle.

Keywords
Pungent
Comforting
Enveloping

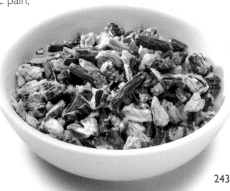

243

Peppermint *(Mentha × piperita)*

A hybrid of Spearmint (*Mentha spicata*; see pp.248–9) and Watermint (*Mentha aquatica*), peppermint is the most pungent mint by far. It has tough, dark stems and serrated green leaves. The essential oil has a cooling, pungent menthol aroma, with clean, sweet top notes.

Plant features: Aromatic herb with lance-shaped leaves

Part of plant used: Leaves

Oil produced in: UK, US

Extraction method: Steam distillation

Safety first
• Peppermint oil is non-toxic.
• This oil is a moderate skin sensitizer: avoid it in baths or massage if you have sensitive skin.

Supporting the spirit
• Peppermint revives depleted energy.
• This oil enhances positivity.

Easing the mind
• To improve poor concentration, vaporize 3 drops Peppermint and 3 drops Rosemary.
• To ease fatigue, take a bath in 2 drops Peppermint and 4 drops Myrtle.

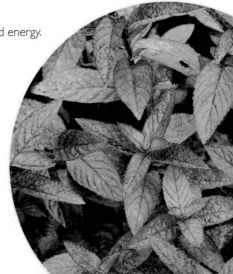

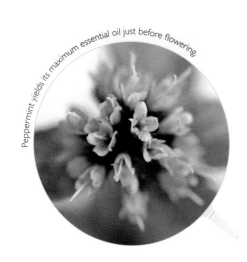

Peppermint yields its maximum essential oil just before flowering.

Keywords

Revitalizing

Energizing

Refreshing

Healing the body

- To soothe abdominal pain caused by indigestion or irritable bowel syndrome, mix Peppermint with Ginger and Nutmeg in a carrier oil (see first blend, right) and apply it clockwise to your abdomen, twice a day.
- To ease nausea, or travel or morning sickness, inhale 2 drops Peppermint on a tissue.
- To relieve sore muscles, mix Peppermint with Rosemary and Black Spruce in a carrier oil (see second blend, right) and apply it to the affected areas at least once a day.
- To reduce pain after sprains or strain, use a cold compress with 2 drops Peppermint and 2 drops Yarrow.

Special blends

Add these essential oils to 20ml/4 tsp carrier oil:

To ease stomach cramps:
2 drops Peppermint,
4 drops Ginger,
4 drops Nutmeg

To soothe aching, painful muscles:
2 drops Peppermint,
4 drops Rosemary,
4 drops Black Spruce

245

Bergamot Mint *(Mentha x piperita var. citrata)*

Bergamot mint is the citrus-scented variety of peppermint (see pp.244–5), its parent plant. It is a vigorous herb with dark green leaves, which have slightly reddish-tinged edges and reddish stems. The essential oil is taken from the leaves and flowering tops just as the plant comes into bloom around midsummer. Bergamot Mint offers a good, fresh alternative to other mints – the oil has a soft, citrusy and lightly minty aroma, with sweet notes.

Safety first

Bergamot Mint oil is non-toxic, non-irritating and non-sensitizing, so is safe for all skin types.

Supporting the spirit

• Bergamot Mint lightens and lifts the heart, gently easing frustration and negativity.

• This oil refreshes inner spontaneity.

Easing the mind

• To ease nervous exhaustion and chronic mental stress, take a bath with 4 drops Bergamot Mint and 2 drops Linaloe Wood.

Plant features: Strongly aromatic herb with dark green leaves

Part of plant used: Leaves and early flowering tops

Oil produced in:
India

Extraction method:
Steam distillation

Special blends

Add these essential oils to 20ml/4 tsp carrier oil:

To relieve bloating, indigestion or a blocked bowel:
4 drops Bergamot Mint, 2 drops Ginger, 4 drops Coriander Seed

To release abdominal tension:
4 drops Bergamot Mint, 4 drops Carrot Seed, 2 drops Neroli

- To help to overcome insomnia caused by an overactive mind, vaporize 3 drops Bergamot Mint and 3 drops Lavender in your bedroom as you go to bed.

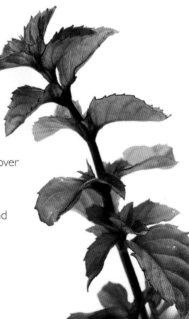

Keywords

Light

Refreshing

Balancing

Healing the body

- To soothe indigestion, wind and constipation, mix Bergamot Mint with Ginger and Coriander Seed in a carrier oil (see first blend, left) and apply it to your abdomen, using clockwise strokes, twice a day.
- To ease acute digestive imbalances linked to emotional stress (which often makes the stomach seize up), mix Bergamot Mint with Carrot Seed and Neroli in a carrier oil (see second blend, left) and apply the blend to your stomach area as often as necessary. Each time, finish by placing a hot-water bottle over the abdomen for extra comfort.
- To ease tension headaches, add 2 drops Bergamot Mint to 5ml/1 tsp carrier oil, and massage the blend into your forehead or temples, or the back of your neck.

Spearmint *(Mentha spicata)*

This herb has vibrant, emerald-green leaves that are soft to touch, and it produces spikes of tiny white flowers in late summer. Spearmint has been a popular herb in British monastery and cottage gardens since medieval times, because it is a valuable remedy for headaches and stomach troubles, as well as soothing the mouth and gums and cleaning the teeth. Fresh leaves make a refreshing herbal tea to settle the digestion. The essential oil is distilled from the leaves and flowering tops in late summer. This oil has a warm, minty and sweet fragrance, with sharp, fresh notes.

Plant features: Garden herb with bright green lance-shaped leaves

Part of plant used: Leaves and flowering tops

Oil produced in: UK

Extraction method: Steam distillation

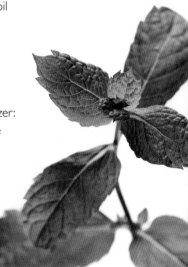

Safety first

- Spearmint oil is non-toxic.
- This oil can be a mild irritant or sensitizer: avoid it in baths or massage if you have sensitive or allergy-prone skin.

Supporting the spirit

- Spearmint soothes and calms fiery emotions, bringing inner tranquillity.

248

• This essential oil encourages inner clarity and inspires new ideas.

Easing the mind
• To even out erratic emotions, bathe with 2 drops Spearmint and 4 drops Orange Leaf.
• To overcome insomnia and bad dreams, vaporize 3 drops Spearmint and 3 drops Lemon beside your bed at night.

Healing the body
• To ease indigestion, stomach cramps and stomach aches, mix Spearmint with Roman Chamomile in a carrier oil (see first blend, right) and apply it to the abdominal area, using clockwise strokes, twice a day.
• To soothe irritable bowel syndrome and chronic, stress-related indigestion, mix Spearmint with Clove Bud and Neroli in a carrier oil (see second blend, right) and rub it into the abdomen, twice a day.
• To support the body's systems during flu, try inhalations and a daily bath with 2 drops Spearmint and 4 drops Cardamom.

Keywords
Warm
Uplifting
Soothing

Special blends

Add these essential oils to 20ml/4 tsp carrier oil:

To soothe stomach pain:
6 drops Spearmint,
4 drops Roman Chamomile *(This blend is especially suitable for children aged over two if you halve the drops.)*

To ease digestive problems:
4 drops Spearmint,
4 drops Clove Bud,
2 drops Neroli

249

Ylang Ylang (*Cananga odorata*)

Meaning "flower of flowers", ylang ylang is a tropical tree that produces its flowers in three different colours — yellow, pink and mauve — all with thick, highly scented petals. The yellow flowers yield the best-quality essential oil; they are distilled slowly, and producers draw off different grades of essential oil at different stages. Look for the best grade — called "Ylang Ylang Extra" — which is extracted first, contains the finest-quality fragrance and has the most therapeutic value in aromatherapy. Ylang Ylang Extra has a very sweet, longlasting, musky aroma, with sharp top notes.

Safety first
- Ylang Ylang oil is non-toxic, non-irritant and non-sensitizing, so is safe for all skin types.
- If you are prone to headaches, this oil has a strong aroma that may trigger an attack.

Supporting the spirit
- Ylang Ylang oil helps to heighten your senses.
- This oil develops the "inner feminine" and a sense of creativity.

Plant features: Tropical tree; heavy-scented blooms

Part of plant used: Yellow flowers

Oil produced in: Madagascar

Extraction method: Steam distillation

Special blends

Add these essential oils to 20ml/4 tsp carrier oil:

To lift mood and ease depression:
2 drops Ylang Ylang, 4 drops Benzoin Resinoid, 4 drops Tangerine

To combat high blood pressure resulting from stress:
2 drops Ylang Ylang, 4 drops Lavender, 4 drops Sweet Orange

Easing the mind

- If you feel anxious and withdrawn, take a bath with 2 drops Ylang Ylang and 4 drops Mandarin.
- To ease depression, mix Ylang Ylang, Benzoin Resinoid and Tangerine in a carrier oil (see first blend, left); apply it to tense areas.

Healing the body

- To raise energy levels and ease physical tiredness associated with pre-menstrual syndrome (PMS), take a bath with 2 drops Ylang Ylang and 4 drops Coriander Seed.
- To clarify greasy or combination skin, apply 2 drops Ylang Ylang, 4 drops Australian Sandalwood and 4 drops Grapefruit in 20g/4 tsp Skin Mousse (see pp.42–3).
- To help to lower stress-related high blood pressure, mix Ylang Ylang with Lavender and Sweet Orange (see second blend, left) and apply it to areas where you store tension, always stroking the blend toward your heart.

Keywords

Sensual

Soothing

Exotic

251

Cistus (Cistus ladaniferus)

Also known as the "rock rose", this bush is intensely aromatic and thrives in the hot, arid climate of the extreme southern Mediterranean and the Middle East. Its aroma comes from a gum that is produced within the plant's leaves and woody tissue. To obtain the gum, the twigs and leaves have to be boiled, then the gum itself is distilled to produce the essential oil. Cistus oil has a longlasting aroma, which lingers on the skin. The fragrance is deep, musky and herbaceous, with sweet notes.

Plant features: Small wild shrub with white flowers

Part of plant used: Gum

Oil produced in: Spain, Middle East

Extraction method: Steam distillation

Safety first
Cistus essential oil is non-toxic, non-irritating and non-sensitizing, so is safe for all skin types.

Supporting the spirit
• Cistus oil purges and heals emotional wounds, allowing new beginnings.
• This essential oil creates a sense of inner peace and harmony.

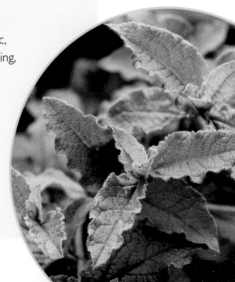

Easing the mind
- To calm shock, sudden emotional trauma or grief, mix Cistus with Neroli and Sweet Orange in a carrier oil (see first blend, right) and gently apply the blend to the areas where you store your tension or trauma.
- To melt frozen emotions, enabling more open communication, take a bath with 2 drops Cistus and 4 drops Rose Geranium.

Healing the body
- To heal wounds, sores, ulcers and skin affected by eczema, mix Cistus with Elemi and German Chamomile in a carrier oil (see second blend, right) and apply it to the affected areas.
- To tone and clarify oily, mature skin with open pores, add 2 drops Cistus, 4 drops Frankincense and 4 drops Grapefruit to 20g/4 tsp Skin Mousse (see pp.42–3) and apply it to your face nightly.
- To soothe the symptoms of candida or thrush, take a bath with 2 drops Cistus and 4 drops Australian Sandalwood.

Keywords

Calming

Warming

Rejuvenating

Special blends

Add these essential oils to 20ml/4 tsp carrier oil:

To soothe the nerves after a shock:
2 drops Cistus, 4 drops Neroli, 4 drops Sweet Orange

To repair sore or infected skin:
2 drops Cistus, 4 drops Elemi, 4 drops German Chamomile

253

Lime *(Citrus aurantifolia)*

Botanists believe that most lime trees originated in Burma and India, and were brought to the Mediterranean region more than a thousand years ago by early Arab traders. Different species of lime tree are also found growing wild in tropical parts of central and northern South America, thanks to the arrival of Spanish and Portuguese settlers in the 16th century. Lime essential oil is expressed from the fruit's peel, which tends to be thinner than lemon or orange peel but is still full of tiny oil-filled sacs. Its aroma is sharp and mouthwateringly bittersweet, as well as citrusy and fresh.

Safety first

- Lime essential oil is non-toxic, non-irritant and non-sensitizing, so is safe for all skin types.
- This oil is highly phototoxic: avoid it in massage if you are going out in the sun.

Supporting the spirit

- Lime oil refreshes inner clarity, enabling better decision-making.

Plant features: Small, evergreen tree

Part of plant used: Fruit peel

Oil produced in: Italy, Spain, Mexico, US

Extraction method: Expression

Special blends

Add these essential oils to 20ml/4 tsp carrier oil:

To ease an overloaded mind:
2 drops Lime,
4 drops Neroli,
4 drops Frankincense

To reduce cellulite and boost the lymph system:
2 drops Lime, 4 drops Juniper Berry, 4 drops Nutmeg

• This oil awakens your sense of inner purpose and boosts energy to move forward.

Easing the mind
• To ease emotional lethargy and listlessness, vaporize 3 drops Lime and 3 drops Bergamot.
• To relieve mental exhaustion, mix Lime with Neroli and Frankincense in a carrier oil (see first blend, left) and rub the blend gently into the skin wherever it soothes you to do so.

Healing the body
• To support the body's systems through colds and flu, try inhalations and daily baths with 2 drops Lime and 4 drops Ginger.
• To lessen cellulite and assist lymphatic drainage, mix Lime with Juniper Berry and Nutmeg in a carrier oil (see second blend, left) and apply it to any areas affected by cellulite, always stroking toward the heart.
• To help with acne and clear oily complexions, add 2 drops Lime, 4 drops Cypress and 4 drops Tinaloe Wood to 20g/4 tsp Skin Mousse (see pp.42–3) and apply it nightly.

Keywords

Revitalizing

Energizing

Refreshing

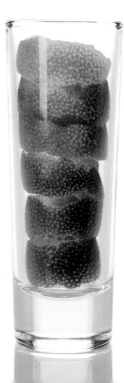

255

Neroli (*Citrus aurantium*)

Neroli (or Orange Blossom) essential oil is distilled from the flowers of the bitter orange tree, which is also the source of Orange Leaf essential oil (see pp.130–31). Neroli is expensive, so suppliers may sell it diluted in Jojoba at "perfume strength" (10 drops essential oil in every 10ml/2 tsp Jojoba). This smells quite strong, and is affordable, but does not give the full benefits of the undiluted oil. Neroli's aroma is rich, sweet and citrusy.

Safety first

Neroli oil is non-toxic, non-irritating and non-sensitizing, so is safe for all skin types.

Supporting the spirit

- Neroli helps to lessen deep-held insecurities.
- This essential oil enables you to feel a complete sense of peace and harmony.

Easing the mind

- To ease insomnia in babies, add 1 drop Neroli to 20ml/4 tsp carrier oil and, after the baby's evening bath, massage it into his or her skin.

Plant features: Evergreen citrus tree

Part of plant used: Blossoms

Oil produced in: Morocco, Egypt

Extraction method: Steam distillation

Special blends

Add these essential oils to 20ml/4 tsp carrier oil:

To ease interrupted or broken sleep:
4 drops Neroli, 4 drops Linaloe Wood, 2 drops Sweet Orange

To support the digestive system through emotional trauma:
4 drops Neroli, 4 drops Bergamot Mint, 2 drops Cardamom

- To calm restless sleep, mix Neroli with Linaloe Wood and Sweet Orange in a carrier (see first blend, left) and apply it to the neck and shoulders nightly.
- To ease shock, place 1 drop Neroli on a tissue and inhale.

Healing the body

- To soothe digestive upsets, mix Neroli with Bergamot Mint and Cardamom in a carrier (see second blend, left) and apply in clockwise abdominal strokes.
- To ease indigestion in children aged between two and ten, add 2 drops Neroli and 2 drops Peppermint to 20ml/4 tsp carrier oil and rub it into the abdomen in a clockwise direction.
- To relieve tiredness during the last trimester of pregnancy, add 2 drops Neroli and 2 drops Sweet Orange to 20ml/4 tsp carrier oil and apply the blend wherever you find it soothing.
- To nourish dry skin, apply 4 drops Neroli, 4 drops Frankincense and 2 drops Rose Otto in 20g/4 tsp Skin Mousse (see pp.42–3).

Keywords

Gentle

Nurturing

Comforting

257

Mandarin (*Citrus reticulata*)

In northern Europe, during the 19th and early 20th centuries, the fruit of the mandarin tree stirred up thoughts of Christmas – the time of year when the fruits arrived from the orchards of the southern Mediterranean. The fruits are similar to tangerines (see pp.230–31), but smaller and with a brighter orange peel. French naturopaths consider mandarins to be extremely beneficial to children and the elderly, because they provide a wealth of vitamin C, but are less acidic than oranges. Mandarin essential oil is available in two types – yellow and green, one expressed from ripe fruit; the other from unripe fruit. Both oils are sweet in fragrance, but yellow Mandarin has a softer aroma, while green Mandarin is slightly fresher. Despite these aromatic differences, the therapeutic uses of the oils are the same.

Safety first

- Mandarin oil is non-toxic, non-irritating and non-sensitizing, so is safe for all skin types.
- Mandarin is not phototoxic, so you can use it on your skin even if you go out in the sun.

Plant features:
Evergreen citrus tree

Part of plant used:
Fruit peel

Oil produced in:
Italy

Extraction method:
Expression

Special blends

Add these essential oils to 20ml/4 tsp carrier oil:

To lift the spirits:
4 drops Mandarin,
2 drops Jasmine
Absolute, 4 drops
Australian Sandalwood

To support convalescence:
4 drops Mandarin,
4 drops Cardamom,
2 drops Bergamot

Supporting the spirit

- Mandarin oil promotes a sense of ease in life.
- This oil boosts creativity, enabling new ideas.

Easing the mind

- To ease depression and emotional stress, mix Mandarin with Jasmine Absolute and Australian Sandalwood in a carrier (see first blend, left) and massage into areas of tension.
- To revive and restore mental energy and zest, vaporize 3 drops Mandarin and 3 drops Lime.

Healing the body

- To support the immune system after a viral infection, mix Mandarin with Cardamom and Bergamot in a carrier (see second blend, left) and apply to your body using gentle strokes.
- To clarify oily skin, apply 4 drops Mandarin, 2 drops Cypress and 4 drops Frankincense in 20g/4 tsp Skin Mousse (see pp.42–3).
- If you are more than four months pregnant, combat stretch marks by massaging 2 drops Mandarin and 2 drops Linaloe Wood in 20ml/4 tsp carrier oil into the abdomen, daily.

Keywords

Light

Refreshing

Revitalizing

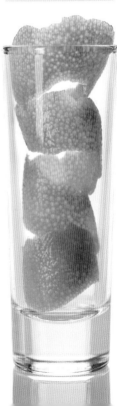

259

Jasmine Absolute *(Jasminum officinale)*

This beautiful, trailing plant produces flowers too delicate for steam distillation – instead, they have to be processed using chemical solvents, giving us an absolute. Jasmine is cultivated in Morocco and Egypt, and also in India, where a species called *Jasminum sambac* yields an absolute even muskier than *Jasminum officinale.* The aroma is rich, floral, very heady, and sweet.

Plant features: Climbing plant with dark green leaves

Part of plant used: Flowers

Oil produced in: Morocco, India, Egypt

Extraction method: Solvent extraction

Safety first

- Jasmine Absolute is non-toxic, but it is a potential skin irritant and sensitizer: avoid it in baths or massage if you have sensitive skin.
- If you are prone to headaches, this oil's strong aroma may trigger an attack.
- Do not use Jasmine Absolute during pregnancy. However, it is safe to use during labour.

Supporting the spirit

- Jasmine Absolute boosts and restores sexual vitality.
- It aids the expression of intimate feelings.

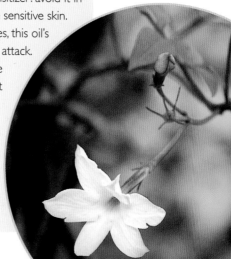

Easing the mind

- To warm cold, withdrawn emotions and to encourage sexual intimacy, mix Jasmine Absolute with Australian Sandalwood and Sweet Orange in a carrier oil (see first blend, right), and apply it anywhere you feel tense.
- To heal chronic emotional stress and withdrawal, take a bath with 2 drops Jasmine Absolute and 4 drops Sweet Orange.

Healing the body

- To regulate menstruation and ease pre-menstrual syndrome (PMS), mix Jasmine Absolute with Agnus Castus and Mandarin in a carrier (see second blend, right) and apply it clockwise to the abdomen in the evening.
- To help the uterus to contract during labour, blend 2 drops Jasmine Absolute and 2 drops Clary Sage in 20ml/4 tsp carrier and ask your partner to massage it into your abdomen.
- To revive mature skin, add 2 drops Jasmine Absolute, 4 drops Frankincense and 4 drops Cistus to 20g/4 tsp Skin Mousse (see pp.42–3) and apply it to your face nightly.

Keywords

Rich

Powerful

Sensual

Special blends

Add these essential oils to 20ml/4 tsp carrier oil:

To warm the emotions:
2 drops Jasmine Absolute, 4 drops Australian Sandalwood, 4 drops Sweet Orange

To regulate menstrual periods and relieve symptoms of PMS:
2 drops Jasmine Absolute, 2 drops Agnus Castus, 6 drops Mandarin

261

Melissa (*Melissa officinalis*)

Also known as lemon balm or bee balm, melissa is named after the Greek word for "bee" – the herb is a magnet to them. The yield of essential oil from the plant's leaves is extremely low, making Melissa one of the most expensive oils of all to buy, and frequently subject to adulteration. True Melissa has a distinct aroma; it is like new-mown grass with sweet, citrusy notes and a hint of earth.

Plant features:
Lemon-scented herb

Part of plant used:
Leaves

Oil produced in:
Spain, France

Extraction method:
Steam distillation

Safety first
- Melissa oil is non-toxic.
- This oil is a mild irritant and sensitizer: avoid it in baths or massage if you have sensitive skin.

Supporting the spirit
- Melissa oil comforts during times of grief.
- This oil helps to alleviate feelings of insecurity and vulnerability.

Easing the mind
- To help to overcome anxiety, shock or panic attacks, take a bath with 2 drops Melissa and 4 drops Lavender.

Special blends

Add these essential oils to 20ml/4 tsp carrier oil:

To calm erratic moods:
2 drops Melissa, 4 drops Roman Chamomile, 4 drops Neroli

To boost the system through chronic fatigue or post-viral conditions:
2 drops Melissa, 4 drops Cubeb Pepper, 4 drops Mandarin

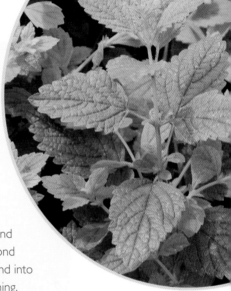

- To stabilize mood swings or calm the emotions, mix Melissa with Roman Chamomile and Neroli in a carrier oil (see first blend, left) and apply it to the skin in long, soothing strokes.

Healing the body

- To soothe symptoms of chronic fatigue and post-viral exhaustion, mix Melissa with Cubeb Pepper and Mandarin in a carrier oil (see second blend, left) and gently rub the blend into your body wherever it feels soothing.
- To ease headaches and migraine, add 2 drops Melissa to 5ml/1 tsp carrier oil and apply it to your forehead, temples or neck.
- To calm indigestion, add 4 drops Melissa, 4 drops Grapefruit and 2 drops Peppermint to 20ml/4 tsp carrier oil and apply it using clockwise abdominal massage, as needed.
- To help to lower stress-related high blood pressure, take a bath containing 2 drops Melissa and 4 drops Neroli.

Keywords
Calming
Cooling
Nurturing

263

Spikenard *(Nardostachys jatamansi)*

Native to the mountains of northern India and Nepal, the spikenard plant has a thick root with a strong and longlasting fragrance. According to the Gospels, Mary Magdalene anointed Christ using spikenard, and its fragrance is said to have filled the house. While it is not possible to say that the spikenard of the Bible is definitely this plant from India, the comments about its powerful aroma suggest that it might have been. In addition, the Romans valued the fragrance as an expensive perfume. Spikenard is an unusual essential oil, with a strong musky, woody and sweet aroma.

Plant features: Aromatic herb with thick root

Part of plant used: Roots

Oil produced in: India, Nepal

Extraction method: Steam distillation

Safety first
This oil is non-toxic, non-irritating and non-sensitizing, so is safe for all skin types.

Supporting the spirit
• Spikenard warms and enhances sexual energy between partners.

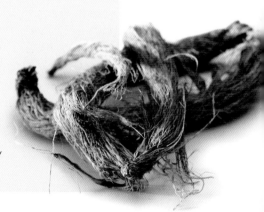

264

• This oil melts frozen emotions and enables the expression of true feelings.

Easing the mind
• To ease shock, grief and panic attacks, mix Spikenard with Rose Otto and Myrrh in a carrier oil (see first blend, right) and apply it to the areas where you tend to store tension.
• To relieve depression and improve low self-image, take a bath with 2 drops Spikenard and 4 drops Rose Geranium.

Healing the body
• To calm palpitations or arrhythmia, mix Spikenard with Immortelle and Neroli in a carrier oil (see second blend, right) and apply it to the chest using circular strokes.
• To soothe eczema or psoriasis, or to heal skin sores, apply 2 drops Spikenard, 4 drops Yarrow and 4 drops Immortelle in 20g/4 tsp Skin Mousse (see pp.42–3) to affected areas.
• To ease digestive imbalance resulting from emotional stress, take a bath with 2 drops Spikenard and 4 drops Orange Leaf.

Keywords

Deep

Sensual

Exotic

Special blends

Add these essential oils to 20ml/4 tsp carrier oil:

To restore calm after emotional trauma:
2 drops Spikenard,
4 drops Rose Otto,
4 drops Myrrh

To regulate the heartbeat:
2 drops Spikenard,
4 drops Immortelle,
4 drops Neroli

265

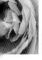

Rose Absolute *(Rosa centifolia)*

Also known as "Rose Maroc", Rose Absolute is usually obtained from the musky-scented flowers of *Rosa centifolia*, an old-fashioned rose with many layers of thin petals (some absolute is also obtained from *Rosa damascena*). *Rosa centifolia* thrives in Morocco and Turkey, where long, hot summers favour maximum flowering. Rose Absolute is produced by using chemical solvents to dissolve the fragrance from the petals; the mixture is then reprocessed to remove the solvents, leaving the absolute, which is orange-red in colour, with an extremely musky, sweet, floral and rich aroma.

Plant features: Prickly bush with scented flowers

Part of plant used: Flowers

Oil produced in: Morocco, Turkey

Extraction method: Solvent extraction

Safety first

Rose Absolute is non-toxic, non-irritating and non-sensitizing, so is safe for all skin types.

Supporting the spirit

- Rose Absolute enriches the "inner feminine".
- It will warm emotional coolness, restoring intimacy.

266

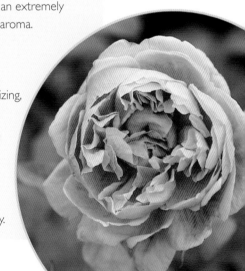

Easing the mind

- To ease hormone-related mood swings, mix Rose Absolute with Fennel and Sweet Orange in a carrier oil (see first blend, right) and apply the blend to your abdomen, using a clockwise motion, every evening.
- To calm feelings of anger and frustration, take a bath with 2 drops Rose Absolute and 4 drops Australian Sandalwood.

Healing the body

- To restore dry, wrinkled or mature skin, apply 2 drops Rose Absolute, 4 drops Frankincense and 4 drops Linaloe Wood in 20g/4 tsp Skin Mousse (see pp.42–3) to your face nightly.
- To overcome tiredness and relieve menopausal hot flashes, blend Rose Absolute, Australian Sandalwood and Agnus Castus in a carrier (see second blend, right) and apply to the body using soothing strokes.
- To soothe eczema or sore skin, add 2 drops Rose Absolute, 4 drops Yarrow and 4 drops Roman Chamomile to 20g/4 tsp Skin Mousse (see pp.42–3) and apply to the affected areas.

Keywords

Rich

Sensual

Beguiling

Special blends

Add these essential oils to 20ml/4 tsp carrier oil:

To ease hormonal mood swings:
2 drops Rose Absolute, 4 drops Fennel, 4 drops Sweet Orange

To boost energy and calm hot flashes:
2 drops Rose Absolute, 4 drops Australian Sandalwood, 4 drops Agnus Castus

267

Rose Otto (*Rosa damascena*)

Otto is the Bulgarian word for "oil" and, since the 17th century, the region around the town of Kazanlik in Bulgaria has been the world's most successful source of Rose Otto essential oil. In the mid-20th century, Bulgarian growers began producing the oil successfully in Turkey, too. Production is labour-intensive: the flowers are handpicked at dawn, when the fragrance is strongest, and it takes around 200 blooms to produce just a few drops of pure oil. Its beautiful fragrance has a honeyed sweetness and subtle fresh, floral top notes.

Plant features:
Old-fashioned bush with irregular growing habit

Part of plant used:
Flowers

Oil produced in:
Bulgaria, Turkey

Extraction method:
Steam distillation

Safety first

This oil is non-toxic, non-irritating and non-sensitizing, so is safe for all skin types.

Supporting the spirit

- Rose Otto nurtures the "inner child".
- This essential oil encourages the expression of unconditional love.

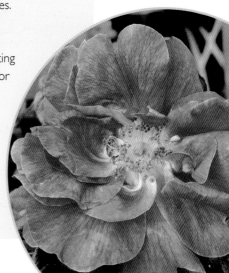

Easing the mind

- To soothe the mood swings of pre-menstrual syndrome (PMS) or the menopause, mix Rose Otto, May Chang and Agnus Castus in a carrier oil (see first blend, right) and massage it into the skin using calming strokes.
- To relieve feelings of grief and sadness, bathe with 2 drops Rose Otto and 4 drops Cistus.

Healing the body

- To soothe dry, sore baby skin, add 1 drop Rose Otto to 20ml/4 tsp carrier oil and gently rub it into the affected areas.
- To help to prevent stretch marks in the second half of pregnancy, mix 2 drops Rose Otto and 2 drops Mandarin in 20ml/4 tsp carrier and apply it daily, using clockwise abdominal strokes.
- To rejuvenate the skin, mix Rose Otto, Neroli and Frankincense in a carrier oil (see second blend, right) and massage into the face, nightly.
- To heal eczema, add 2 drops Rose Otto and 2 drops Lavender to 20g/4 tsp Skin Mousse (see pp.42–3); apply it to the affected areas.

Keywords

Gentle

Nurturing

Uplifting

Special blends

Add these essential oils to 20ml/4 tsp carrier oil:

To balance hormone-related mood swings:
2 drops Rose Otto,
4 drops May Chang,
4 drops Agnus Castus

To restore dry or mature skin:
2 drops Rose Otto,
4 drops Neroli, 4 drops Frankincense

Linden Blossom Absolute (*Tilia europea*)

This unusual absolute comes from the tiny yellow, honey-scented blossoms of the linden blossom tree. The flowers are handpicked, then processed using solvents to make a sticky, semi-solid absolute. You can buy Linden Blossom either liquefied with alcohol or in its semi-solid state. If you buy it semi-solid, add 10ml/2 tsp Jojoba to the absolute, and then place the container in a small bowl of hot water and stir until the absolute dissolves. The fragrance is hay-like, with slight citrus and earth tones.

Safety first

- Linden Blossom Absolute is non-toxic.
- This absolute may be an irritant or sensitizer: avoid it in baths or massage if you have sensitive or allergy-prone skin.

Supporting the spirit

- Linden Blossom Absolute centres inner awareness, bringing a sense of tranquillity.
- This absolute protects us from negative influences, such as others' anger, giving a sense of being nurtured and protected.

Plant features: Tall deciduous tree with heart-shaped leaves

Part of plant used: Flowers

Oil produced in: France

Extraction method: Solvent extraction

Special blends

Add these essential oils to 20ml/4 tsp carrier oil:

To alleviate anxiety:
2 drops Linden Blossom Absolute, 4 drops May Chang, 4 drops Cubeb Pepper

To relieve indigestion or stomach upsets:
2 drops Linden Blossom Absolute, 4 drops Sweet Orange, 4 drops Coriander Seed

270

Easing the mind

- To ease mental anxiety, mix
  Linden Blossom Absolute with
  May Chang and Cubeb Pepper
  in a carrier oil (see first blend,
  left) and apply it wherever it
  feels comforting to do so.
- To soothe stress-related
  headaches or migraines, add
  2 drops Linden Blossom Absolute to
  5ml/1 tsp carrier oil and massage the
  blend into your forehead or neck.

Healing the body

- To ease stress-related indigestion or stomach
  trouble, mix Linden Blossom Absolute
  with Sweet Orange and Coriander Seed
  (see second blend, left) and apply it to the
  abdomen, using clockwise strokes, twice a day.
- To support liver function, especially the
  digestion of fatty foods, add 2 drops Linden
  Blossom, 1 drops Grapefruit and 4 drops
  Fennel to 20ml/4 tsp carrier oil and apply it
  to the abdomen, clockwise, twice a day.

Keywords

Soothing

Uplifting

Subtle

271

Vanilla Absolute (*Vanilla planifolia*)

The vanilla pod comes from a climbing vine related to the orchid. This vine produces trumpet-shaped white flowers, which are usually pollinated by hummingbirds, but are sometimes hand-pollinated by farmers. After pollination, the plant takes about nine months to form the vanilla pod, which, when processed using solvent extraction, yields Vanilla Absolute. This is a sticky, semi-solid mass that needs to be liquefied. Add 10ml/2 tsp Jojoba oil to your pot of Vanilla Absolute, then place it in a small bowl of hot water, stirring until the absolute dissolves. The aroma is soft and resiny, with sweet balsamic notes. Vanilla Absolute is often subject to adulteration – check with your supplier that their product is pure.

Plant features: Climbing plant with large flowers

Part of plant used: Pods (beans)

Oil produced in: Mexico, Madagascar

Extraction method: Solvent extraction

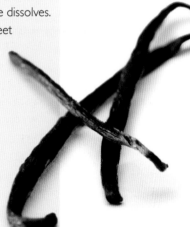

Safety first
• Vanilla Absolute is non-toxic and non-irritant.
• This absolute can be sensitizing: avoid it in baths or massage if you have sensitive skin.

272

Supporting the spirit
• Vanilla Absolute promotes a sense of inner peace and relaxation.
• This absolute enhances intimacy.

Easing the mind
• To deeply relax the mind after a period of emotional stress, mix Vanilla Absolute with Neroli and Orange Leaf in a carrier oil (see first blend, right) and apply it to your body in whichever way you find soothing.
• To soothe away panic attacks, and relieve shock and anxiety, take a bath with 2 drops Vanilla Absolute and 4 drops Linaloe Wood.
• To warm cold feelings and enhance sexual energy, mix Vanilla Absolute with Jasmine Absolute and Sweet Orange in a carrier oil (see second blend, right) and rub it gently into your skin wherever you feel tension.

Healing the body
• Aromatherapists tend not to use Vanilla Absolute to overcome physical conditions; it is primarily a soothing and sensual fragrance.

Keywords

Sensual

Exotic

Alluring

Special blends

Add these essential oils to 20ml/4 tsp carrier oil:

To alleviate emotional overload and calm the mind:
2 drops Vanilla Absolute, 4 drops Neroli, 4 drops Orange Leaf

To enhance intimacy:
2 drops Vanilla Absolute, 2 drops Jasmine Absolute, 6 drops Sweet Orange

273

Violet Leaf Absolute (*Viola odorata*)

A tender flower with purple blooms and a cool, soft scent, violet grows best in fresh, moist and shady locations, such as woodland. In Western herbal medicine, violet flowers and leaves are traditional remedies for lung conditions, coughs and viruses; and the fresh, crushed leaves provide a skin antiseptic for cuts and wounds. Violet Leaf Absolute has a strong, leafy aroma, tempered by sweet, floral hints.

Plant features: Small wild flower with heart-shaped leaves

Part of plant used: Leaves

Oil produced in: France

Extraction method: Solvent extraction

Safety first
- Violet Leaf Absolute is non-toxic.
- This absolute can be an irritant or sensitizer: avoid it in baths or massage if you have hypersensitive skin.

Supporting the spirit
- Violet Leaf Absolute soothes fiery emotions.
- This absolute can awaken awareness of the subtle body and its energy.

Easing the mind
- To soothe nervous exhaustion, mix Violet Leaf Absolute with Spikenard and Mandarin in a

Special blends

Add these essential oils to 20ml/4 tsp carrier oil:

To soothe a depleted nervous system:
2 drops Violet Leaf Absolute, 2 drops Spikenard, 6 drops Mandarin

To clarify oily skin:
2 drops Violet Leaf Absolute, 4 drops Rose Geranium, 4 drops Lemon

274

carrier oil (see first blend, left) and gently rub the blend into your skin, focusing on areas of tension.
- To ease frontal stress headaches, add 2 drops Violet Leaf Absolute to 5ml/1 tsp carrier oil and apply it gently to your forehead.

Healing the body
- To heal wounds or ulcers, or relieve eczema or skin infections, add 2 drops Violet Leaf Absolute, 4 drops Yarrow and 4 drops Myrrh to 20g/4 tsp Skin Mousse (see pp.42–3) and apply it to the affected areas.
- To clarify oily skin, mix Violet Leaf Asbolute, Rose Geranium and Lemon in a carrier (see second blend, left) and apply to the face.
- To ease chesty or painful coughs, add 2 drops Violet Leaf Absolute, 4 drops Myrtle and 4 drops Himalayan Cedarwood to 20ml/4 tsp carrier oil and massage the blend into the chest every morning and evening.

Keywords
Soft
Calming
Cooling

275

For reference

Glossary

absolute an aromatic extract obtained using chemical solvents

antidepressant helps to combat poor self-esteem and depression

antifungal fights fungal infections, such as athlete's foot

antiviral fights viral infections, such as flu

blend a combination of essential oils and a carrier oil

carrier oil a vegetable oil used as a base for massage to dilute essential oils so that they are safe to apply to the skin

chemotype an essential oil produced from a plant species in a particular geographical location that influences the oil's chemical balance

clarify to remove excess oil and surface dirt from the skin's upper layers

dilution precise percentages of essential oils in carrier oil calculated so that the oils may be used safely

distillation the process of using water and/or steam to remove aromatic particles from plant tissue

essential oil a natural plant fragrance

obtained by distillation or expression from a single botanical source

expression the process of pressing essential oil out of citrus fruit peel

fatty acids found in vegetable oils; chains of molecules with skin-softening traits

gum a sticky mass that oozes from the wood of certain trees and bushes

mucous membranes the moist, delicate linings of the mouth, digestive tract and genito-urinary area

perfume "notes" different levels of fragrance that combine in a perfume to make the most complete scent; they are denoted in perfumery as:
- **top** the blend's freshest fragrance
- **middle** the blend's balancing scents
- **base** the aroma's longlasting notes

perfume "terms" descriptive words used in perfumery to denote particular fragrances, such as:
- **balsamic** sweet and slightly spicy
- **camphoraceous** medicinal-smelling
- **citrus** sharp, like lemon
- **earthy** like turned soil

- **floral** sweet and rosy
- **woody** like wood chippings

post-viral fatigue the term used to describe symptoms that linger after a viral illness, including tiredness

rhizome a fleshy root, as in ginger

skin type a way to describe the tone and appearance of skin, in particular:
- **normal** perfectly balanced, not too oily or dry, with a silky appearance
- **combination** with oily patches across the brow, down the sides of the nose and on the chin, with dry cheeks
- **oily** greasy, with a shiny appearance

stimulant something that increases local circulation so that the skin glows pink

vasodilation the opening up of the blood vessels to allow better blood-flow

Bibliography

Battaglia, S., *The Complete Guide to Aromatherapy* (2nd ed.), International Centre of Holistic Aromatherapy (Brisbane, Australia), 2003

Davis, P., *Aromatherapy – an A–Z*, DANI (London, UK), 2007

Harding, Jennie, *Secrets of Aromatherapy*, Dorling Kindersley (London, UK), 2000

Harding, Jennie, *Aromatherapy Massage for You*, DBP (London, UK), 2005

Harding, Jennie, *Incense*, Polair Publishing (London, UK), 2005

Harding, Jennie, *Live Better Aromatherapy*, DBP (London, UK), 2006

Harding, Jennie, *Stress Management*, Hodder Arnold (London, UK), 2006

Lawless, Julia, *The Illustrated Encyclopaedia of Essential Oils*, Element Books (London, UK), 2002

Rose, Jeanne, *375 Essential Oils and Hydrosols*, Frog (Berkeley, CA, USA), 1999

Schnaubelt, Kurt, *Advanced Aromatherapy*, Healing Arts Press (Rochester, VT, USA), 1995

Tisserand, Robert, *The Art of Aromatherapy*, CW Daniels (Saffron Walden, Sussex, UK), 1977

Tisserand, Robert, and Balacs, Tony, *Essential Oil Safety*, Churchill Livingstone (London, UK), 1999

Useful addresses

Contact these associations
to find out about professional
aromatherapy training or how
to contact a qualified
practitioner near you.

___

**IFA (International Federation
of Aromatherapists)**
61–63 Churchfield Rd,
London, W3 6AY, UK
Tel: +44 (0) 20 8992 9605
Fax: +44 (0) 20 8992 7983
Website: www.ifaroma.org
Email: office@ifaroma.org

**IFPA (International Federation
of Professional Aromatherapists)**
82 Ashby Rd, Hinckley,
Leicestershire,
LE10 1SN, UK
Tel: +44 (0) 1455 637 987
Website: www.ifparoma.org
Email: admin@IFPAroma.org

**CTHA (Complementary Therapists
Association; ITEC therapists)**
PO BOX 6955,
Towcester, NN12 6WZ, UK
Tel: +44 (0) 844 779 8899
Fax: +44 (0) 844 779 8898
Website: www.complementary.assoc.org.uk
Email: info@complementary.assoc.org.uk

**The National Association for Holistic
Aromatherapy (NAHA)**
3327 W. Indian Trail Rd PMB 144,
Spokane, WA 99208, USA
Tel: +1 509 325 3419
Fax: +1 509 325 3479
Website: www.naha.org
Email: info@naha.org

**International Federation of
Aromatherapists (IFA) Australian Branch**
PO BOX 215 Burwood,
NSW 1805, Australia
Tel +61 (0) 2 9715 6622
Fax +61 (0) 2 9715 5922
Website: www.ifa.org.au
Email info@ifa.org.au

Index

283

Acknowledgments

Heartfelt thanks to the team at DBP – especially to Kelly, Judy, Justin and Jules – for all their hard work on this book. **Jennie Harding**

Picture credits

Picture Research by Susannah Stone

The publisher would like to thank the following photographic libraries for permission to reproduce their material. Any errors or omissions are entirely unintentional and the publishers will, if informed, make amendments in future editions of this book:

Page 13 Altrendo Images/Getty Images; **24** Dorling Kindersley/Getty Images; **37** Shaun Egan/Getty Images; **55** Japack Photo/Photolibrary; **81** Victoria Gomez/Flowerphotos; **83** David Murray/DK Images; **85** Douglas Peebles/Corbis; **91** Garden Picture Library/ Photolibrary; **98** Bob Gibbon/Science Photo Library; **101** Laurie Campbell/NHPA; **108** Steffen Hauser/Botanikfoto; **116** Pascal Goetgheluck/Science Photo Library; **132** Garden Picture Library/Photolibrary; **139** Carol Sharp/Flowerphotos; **145** Botanica/Photolibrary; **151** Jerry Mason/Science Photo Library; **165** Rod Planck/ NHPA; **171** Maria Mosolova/Flowerphotos; **175** Bsip/Photolibrary; **187** Andrew Lawson Photography; **189** Garden Picture Library/Photolibrary; **190** Dave Watts/ NHPA; **191** Geoff Kidd/Science Photo Library; **192** Cristine Pedrazzini/Science Photo Library; **208** Daniel Heuelin/NHPA; **211** Garden Picture Library/Photolibrary; **213** Steffen Hauser/Botanikfoto; **217** David Nunuk/Science Photo Library; **220** Botanica/ Photolibrary; **223** Andy Crawford & Steve Gorton/DK Images; **239** Andrew Lawson Photography; **251** Deni Bown; **268** Garden Picture Library/Photolibrary

Publisher's acknowledgments

The publisher would like to thank the following people for their help with this book: Jules Hayward at the Royal Botanic Gardens, Kew, and Jan Wells and all at Essentially Oils Ltd, who supplied vaporizers and oils for the photoshoots.

Essentially Oils Ltd
8–10 Mount Farm,
Churchill, Chipping Norton,
Oxfordshire,
OX7 6NP, UK
Tel +44 (0) 1608 659 544
Fax +44 (0) 1608 659 566
Website: www.essentiallyoils.com
Email: sales@essentiallyoils.com

Royal Botanic Gardens, Kew
Kew Green,
Richmond,
Surrey,
TW9 3AB, UK
Tel +44 (0) 20 8332 5655
Fax +44 (0) 20 8332 5197
Website: www.kew.org
Email: info@kew.org

About the Royal Botanic Gardens, Kew

The Royal Botanic Gardens, Kew, has been collecting plants – both living and preserved – for nearly 250 years. The focus of interest is on wild or native species of plants from around the world. If your taste is for the more flamboyant hybrids or cultivars, Kew may not be for you, but if you are interested in native plants and their properties, Kew Gardens is "ground zero" of the plant kingdom. Some 35,000 different species can be seen in the gardens and glasshouses, making the UK's TW9 the most plant biodiverse postcode in the world. Please come to visit.